WE ARE WHAT WE EAT AND DO:

PRACTICAL BIBLICAL PRINCIPLES FOR A HEALTHY ZIMBABWEAN IN DIASPORA

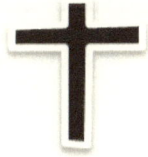

Dr. Natsai L. Zhou Ph.D.

Recipes by: Batiraishe Zhou-Griffin

Sophia Zhou

Cover photo by Natsai L. Zhou PhD

We Are What We Eat And Do: Practical Biblical Principles For A Healthy Zimbabwean In Diaspora

ISBN-13: 978-1500183349
ISBN-10: 1500183342
Category: Christian, Nutrition, Health, Zimbabwean, Diaspora
Library of Congress Cataloging-in-Publication Data

Printed in the United States of America

DEDICATION

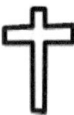

To Jesus Christ God Almighty- I give you honor and all the
glory, for without you this book would not be possible.
Only you truly know the depths and breath of my journey.

**My Zimbabwean Family on the Prayer-Line (and Mainini vangu
Mbuya VaNathaniel)**-without your willing to listen to what I
share; and your support, I would not have an audience.
NDINOTENDA!

**Prayer Line Pastors, Preachers, Singers, Bible Readers and
Facilitators:** For the time you take to spiritually feed us and
keep the Prayer Line going, you are my life line. Thank you,
kubvuma kutumwa naShe.

**My parents: Ambassador Dr. Sifas and Mrs. Sophia Zhou (Mma
Bathu) -** Mom thank you for your love and time you take to
prepare all those wonderful meals for us. Dad, thank you for
you all the funny stories and jokes you share during dinner
time. Thank you both for giving me life, love, support; and
always believing in me and praying for me. You are the wind
beneath my wings, and I am honored to have you as my
parents.

ACKNOWLEDGEMENTS

MmaBathu (Mom) – Thankful for being my Google-live, and the recipes.

Bati Zhou-Griffin- So grateful for all the time you put in the recipes, actually going out to shop and trying them out to see what/how it would work in Diaspora. Grateful for your contribution to the book.

Mrs Anyiwo- Infinitely appreciative for being generous with your time, priceless editorial advice and feedback; but most of all for the words of encouragement and your vision.

Rati Zhou- For believing in me, always.

Tinei Zhou- For saying this was a great book but mostly for my *muroora* **Sharon Zhou** for taking the time to read, and thoroughly enjoy the first 3 chapters, and providing encouraging feedback.

Vushe Zhou- For your contagious laugh as you read some excerpts from the book and your nostalgic renditions.

Pastor Marvelous (WOD President) - For encouraging me with Ps. 37:23 when things seemed to go wrong telling me to *"keep walking."*

Sister's Keepers- My Nashville crew keeping me on my toes: **Rev. Eva. Mudambanuki**- calling me at 6am to says *"Dr. Zhou you need to finish that book!"* **Violet Mashingaidze**-*"I can't wait to read the whole book"* (thank you for the laptop back up), **Davidzo Gambiza-** *"How far are you with the book?"* & **Thandi Thondlana-** *"Finish that book so we can go back to zumba & hiking"*

Professor Lupafya, Rufaro Katedza, & Thandi Mamutse- My God given sister-friends. Always there, believing in me; praying, laughing, and crying with me.

Cherie Archer: For last minute- pagination, running heads!! And being that 3rd eye! Much appreciated!

Table of Contents

PREFACE

As a Christian and a healthcare practitioner, I have always sought out a platform that I could combine God's given profession and what I belief to be my purpose in life; to serve His people. About four years ago, I started attending two Prayer Lines– (*Church isinia madziro*) one hosted by Pastor Masuka (known to most as Sekuru Masuka), and the other by Reverend Mudambanuki. On these teleconferences, Zimbabweans living outside Zimbabwe (in Diaspora) are blessed with sermons from anointed Zimbabwean women and men of God. They provide us with an amazing opportunity to worship, pray, and praise the Lord in a familiar environment. Two years ago, I was asked to join Sekuru Masuka's Patsime Life Class Team to provide health related issues presentations. This book is inspired by many Zimbabweans who listen to these presentations and request notes from the lessons presented. I give God the honor for allowing me the opportunity to continue using my profession on this Christian podium.

I would like to express that this book does not by any means represent every Zimbabwean in Diaspora's lived experience. Illustrations used are solely an attempt to relate discussed issues in a practical and familiar manner.

I am by no means a Pastor or Preacher. Neither did I attend theological school. Verses incorporated in this book are based on my understanding of the Word and the way I incorporate it in my life. During the presentations, one of the great things that God continues to teach me is that I am also my own audience, and from the conception of this book to its birth, I have been the greatest learner/student.

It is therefore, my wish and prayer that whoever reads this book is able to say, "Yes, I did learn something, and I intend to make some healthy lifestyle changes, with God's help."

INTRODUCTION

We Are What We Eat And Do: Practical Biblical Principles For A Healthy Zimbabwean In Diaspora **is book 1 of 2.** It is written to address eating habits and behaviors that may affect our health as Zimbabweans in Diaspora. It is more applicable to those of us living in the Western and Eastern world, where we are more challenged accessing home than those in Africa. For some of us, maybe easy to go online and find answers to any health/nutrition question, or call our healthcare providers, our pastors, or even our mothers. However, for those who might not have the opportunity, this book is written for easy access to some of the questions that might be lingering in our minds about food, health, and how all this connects to the Word of God. Therefore, Bible scriptures (NIV *ne BHAIBHERI*), sermons, review of literature, and yes, discussions with mom are applied to help understand our bodies and nutrition using Biblical principles. It is my greatest pleasure to say that today even the secular world is adopting healthier ways of living that have Biblical foundation. As Christians, our attitudes toward the food we eat, our behaviors, and our bodies should include Biblical insights. In this book, I will strive to connect selected passages of scriptures to our nutrition, life styles, and health.

Book 2

Upcoming **Book 2** will address the connection between what we eat, how we view ourselves, and our lifestyles, including exercise, to related diseases/illnesses. Biblical principles will continue to be applied as our foundation of our practice.

CHAPTER ONE

EXODUS: *KUBUDA*

"I am God, the God of your father," he said. "Do not be
afraid to go down to Egypt, for I will make you into a
great nation there. I will go down to Egypt with you"
(Genesis 46: 3-4a).

Nothing God ever does is a mistake. It is always for our own good. God moves us to certain places at a certain time for a certain reason. It is not by luck or accident that the Lord allowed us to leave *(kubuda)* our motherland and lead us to a place where we are today. With that in mind, God never left us alone through our journey, although from time to time we might have left Him. Wherever God moves us, He also promises to make us a great nation because he has the best intentions for us and thus, He has plans for everyone to prosper and not to be harmed:

> *"For I know the plans I have for you," declares the*
> *LORD, "plans to prosper you and not to harm you,*
> *Plan to give you hope and a future" (Jeremiah 29:11).*

To achieve the plans God has for us, we need to meet our responsibilities. Besides believing in His promises, our responsibilities requires us to be physically, mentally, and spiritually equipped in order to achieve the greatness that the Lord has in store for us. During a church sermon, I once heard my pastor explain the word "responsibility," saying it meant that we have the "ability" to "respond." That means we do have the capability to answer to our call, but we should to be healthy beings to do so.

Our God was the same yesterday, is the same today and will not change tomorrow. Just like God promised Jacob and Abram yesterday, He promises to stand for us today and will continue to do so for the next generation tomorrow:

> *The LORD had said to Abram, "Go from your country,*
> *your people and your father's household to the land I will*
> *show you. I will make you into a great nation, and I will*
> *bless you; I will make your name great and you will be a*
> *blessing" (Genesis 12: 1-2).*

God desires for us to be blessed. None of us should take this promise lightly. No matter who or what we were back home, this promise is for all of us wherever we are. Being in Diaspora, while missing home, we are confronted with many challenging barriers such as cultural and lifestyle differences; as well as a variety of food types. This is when we need the living Word of God to guide us. Most of the time, it seems easier for us to ask for God's guidance when dealing with sickness, loss of a loved one, having financial and relationship problems, or when we are just in plain trouble. However, not many of us consider seeking Godly guidance when dealing with nutritional issues or what we should be putting in our bodies. Yet, food though created good, can be a root of many health issues. There are so many Christian seminars offered on matters such as what God says about our finances, marriage, death, purpose in life, how to deal with work issues, or even manage emotions. We are even provided Biblical verses to encourage us with these different issues. But what about what God says about food, our bodies, and health? Are there Biblical principles we can use to help us stay healthy as well as prevent illness and diseases that are food related?

Health issues can be very complicated, even more so when in a foreign land where we are exposed to different foods, eating habits, and behaviors. So many things factor into what is considered healthy, and these factors can be perceived differently by each one of us. While teaching a healthcare course, I once asked my students what it meant to be healthy. Responses included:

"Being disease free"

"Not feeling sick"

"Being able to work and take care of family"

"Looking fit or in shape"

"Eating well"

"Exercising"

From these statements, one can conclude that if one does not have a disease, is not feeling sick, is able to work and take care of one's family, is looking good, eating well, or exercising, one is healthy. In addition, it appears that any of these characteristics can be used exclusively or in combination to describe a healthy person. As a healthcare provider, I can say that the above descriptions barely scratch the surface of the picture of health. Unfortunately, it is possible to still have an illness harboring our bodies and not feel sick until it is too late. It is also possible to be in good shape or fit and not be able to work. Furthermore, the definition of healthy eating and exercising can be misleading if one is not informed of its meaning. Regrettably, there are times when we might think that we are eating healthy only to discover the contrary.

The phrase "you are what you eat" should not be taken lightly for what we see is not necessarily what is going on inside the body at which we are looking. Therefore, beloved, in this book it's my

> *Prayer that in all respects you may prosper and be in*
> *good health, just as your soul prospers (3 John 1:2).*

What I now know

In this chapter what I found most interesting is:

_____

_____

_____

_____

_____

~~~~

From this chapter I intend to do the following toward healthier eating:

_____

_____

_____

_____

_____

CHAPTER TWO

GENESIS: *MA VAMBO*

God saw all that he had made, and it was very good ...
(Genesis 1: 31a).

Yes, it was good it was very good. In the beginning, *(kumavambo)* back in our past, on any given Zimbabwe Saturday afternoon, in any township neighborhood, one could hear children's laughter and shouting as they ran around playing and chasing each other across the yards and lawns outside. The back or front yards consisted of an array of vegetables, onions, carrots, tomatoes to name a few; and rows of fruit trees bursting with sweet mangoes, paw-paws, bright yellow lemons and juicy oranges, which were watered faithfully. Children would stop playing *pada* (hop scotch) long enough to pick fresh, organic, healthy, ripe *mahabrosi* (mulberries) or juicy mangoes off the back yard tree and snack.

In a little while, the mother would be heard calling one of the kids to go and buy *huku* for *usavi* (chicken for dinner) from the neighbors who raise chicken. The father would be sitting on the veranda drinking a cold bottle of Fanta reading the paper, while *sisi* (helper) went to the garden to pluck a handful of green leaves of rape or *kovho*, tomatoes, and onions.

WE ARE WHAT WE EAT AND DO:

At the same time in the country, kids would also be heard running around in the dust kicking a plastic made soccer ball or pushing self-made toy cars from a wire coat hanger, before the mother called out for them to chase after and catch one of the chickens to be slaughtered for dinner. She would be making her way to the garden to pick up some green leaves of *muboora* (pumpkin leaves) or *munyevhe* (spider flower leaves). After coming from *kumunda* (ploughing in the fields), the father would be sitting under a baobab tree shade drinking some home brewed *maheu* (mealie-meal fermented drink).

In both these families, after a little while, the mouthwatering aroma of meat browning in unison with chopped garden picked onions and tomatoes would soon find its way to everyone's nostrils; including the neighbors' or passers-by who would soon know that the family was having chicken for dinner.

The scenarios described above could have taken place in anyone of our lives when we were growing up back in Zimbabwe. Years later, we got on a flight that left our motherland underneath a blanket of white clouds headed for greener pastures. No matter the reason, each one of us left Zimbabwe: be it to pursue higher education, escape political, and economic hardships or come to visit; most of us stayed abroad longer than we anticipated. Most of us left home believing the same covenant God made to the Israelites - to be blessed. On that same promise we packed our bags and emigrated from Zimbabwe to the Western or even Eastern lands. As Charles Dickens put it in *A Tale of Two Cities:* "It was the best of times, it was the worst of times" that prompted us to leave our green homeland for "greener pastures" intending to return back home to improve our lives as well as those of our families. Five, ten even twenty years later, we find ourselves still in Diaspora, still working to put together our lives here as well as support those back home.

As we continue in this existence, little by little, we start adopting the ways of our new environment, sometimes forgetting some of our native ways. For some, it happens without much attempt or awareness; for others, it occurs with some added effort to change. Anytime we change our lifestyles, on some level our belief system is also compromised. This may be manifested in the manner in which we behave, raise our children, how we think, and even what we eat. Depending on the changes we make, our lives can be affected in ways we may not immediately see but can alter our health in the long run.

As we recollect our childhood playing outside the house, we get a sense of sadness as we hardly see that in Diaspora. We also grew up eating natural, freshly picked fruits and vegetables, and not canned or even frozen. For the most part, breakfast options consisted of *bota rine dovi* (hot porridge with peanut butter), not greasy breakfast sandwiches, or sugary pop-tarts and cold cereal. Lunch and dinner plates almost always had a starch (*sadza*), protein as peanut butter or beans (*nyama, dovi*) and freshly picked vegetables (*murivo*) to make relish. In between meals, mostly lunch and dinner, we were called to come in and wash off some dirt from our feet and hands and get a snack of bread with jam, a fruit or a drink of *maheu*.

Growing up, almost every family had some kind of help around the house. Help consisted of cooking, cleaning, taking care of the children and outside work such as gardening. It really did not matter to which societal class we belonged in order to be able to have help around the house. For those who could afford to pay someone, they employed a maid (*sisi vebasa*) and garden boy. Those who could not afford to hire anyone, got help from extended family members who came to stay with them as reciprocity for the assistance they provided. Either way, most people grew up with almost a full house and some kind of support system around the house. If both parents worked outside the home, there was a person who made sure there was hot food on the table for everyone at each meal. Fathers and mothers would take to work home cooked meals for lunch.

The hot served meals were freshly prepared from natural raised and prepared meat and produce. If store bought, the meat, which was usually chicken or beef, was back yard raised. *Sadza* was made from mealie-meal from corn, which was mostly store bought. Some corn was purchased from the mill (*mugaiwa*), where it was freshly ground and not over processed. *Sadza* also came from different types of *mugaiwa*, stone ground grain-millet such as *mapfunde, mhunga, rukweza* or *zviyo*, which could also be served with store bought lacto or *mage* (curdled sour milk).

What I now know

In this chapter what I found most interesting is:

_____

_____

_____

_____

_____

~~~~

From this chapter I intend to do the following toward healthier eating:

_____

_____

_____

_____

_____

CHAPTER THREE

DIASPORA: IN THE WILDERNESS

You shall walk in all the way that the Lord your God
has commanded you, that you may live, and that it may
go well with you, and that you may live long in the land
that you shall possess (Deuteronomy 5:33).

When we landed in the lands beyond, most of us did not know what to expect. Even having heard about life in Diaspora from those who had migrated before us, the reality was still surreal. It was like a wilderness. The environment and culture were obvious differences. Far gone were the days when families had helpers in their homes. Today in Diaspora not many of us can afford hiring a helper to assist with the cooking, cleaning, as well as taking care of the children, let alone with yard work. Most mothers who work outside the home are similarly faced with doing as much work in the home. Balancing trying to get the children ready for school in the morning and getting ready for work, working late hours or odd hours (3pm to 11pm, 11pm to 7 am, 7pm to 7am) mothers seldom have time or opportunity to be home with the family. Because of those odd hours, mothers simply cannot put hot meals on the table for dinner every night. Technology and living arrangements have also made kids playing outside an ancient behavior as many live in apartments without access to play yards.

We now find ourselves sitting in the homes bought from our hard-earned money, surrounded by comfortable environments in the Diaspora as we get accustomed to the life of abundance and wide choices in grocery stores. When we go grocery shopping in regular stores, we are greeted by robust selections of processed and unprocessed, light, full fat, pre-cooked, frozen, sweet savory food products that line vast brightly lit grocery store shelves baiting us to buy one and get the other one for free. As we drive back from work tired, we zoom past fast food restaurants, some tempting us by advertising new low-calorie, low-fat meals with sugar-free drinks.

When we try our best to eat healthy organic foods, we soon find out that our pockets cannot stretch that far for that long. Even when they can, the scarcity of foods we used to eat back home is vast. We also quickly find out that the products readily available to us fill our stomachs with empty nutrition wreaking havoc on the heart and other vital organs while expanding our bodies. All of the choices of what to eat, stacked up amidst the hustle and bustle lifestyles most of us live in the Diaspora, leave us with no viable options except to put our health on the back burner (pun intended). We work, go to school, work, attend to family matters here and in Zimbabwe, do *madouble* (double shifts),

WE ARE WHAT WE EAT AND DO:

pick up kids from extracurricular activities, and sports, and work again, we are just too busy! We quickly learn that we can't do it all because we have no help! Who will bathe the children and do their hair, who will wash and fold the laundry and vacuum, who will go and buy groceries, and who will cook *sadza*? We are in the Diaspora wilderness!

Subsequently, we sit back and think of the environment most of us were blessed to grow up in. Back then, we never stopped to think about the nutritious valued of the food in front of us and took life events as they came. As we ate our food, we also did not realize to what extent the *muriwo* (fresh leafy greens), the stone ground unprocessed corn and the naturally raised chicken, goats or cattle were nourishing to our health. In Diaspora low-fat-low-calorie commercials remind us every day of the unhealthy food surrounding us. Not everyone has a big enough yard to keep chicken or grow fruits and vegetables, let alone have time to tend to them. Not many of us are able to afford to get help to tend the chickens, the garden or the orchard if we own them. The invasion of nostrils with aroma of fried onions and browning meat is not an everyday occurrence anymore and the voice of *sisi* calling everyone to come inside and eat together has somehow been silenced. Sisi, whose role was and is still a Godsend, added more hours to the normal 24-hour day that we now wish we had by making sure the meat was defrosting in a timely manner, expertly cut up and cooked with fresh vegetables and the starch of the day.

Some of us take good health for granted until we start to lose it and the aches and pains set in; by then we are caught in a cycle of prescriptions, medical equipment, and wheelchairs. No matter what is going on in our lives today, we should strive to live based on God's commands and His good will for us. If we follow His commands to walk in His ways, we will live well and longer and all will go well with us in this land to which He led us. These commands were said in view of the different foods, behaviors and lifestyles we would potentially face. After all, the One who created us knows what is best for us:

> *Before I formed you in the womb I knew you, before you were born I set you apart…(Jeremiah 1:5a).*

Attitudes toward food, our bodies, activities

By no means does this book imply that everything we did back home was according to God's commands, fruitful, and healthy; or that everything we encounter in Diaspora is contrary. We certainly could benefit from adopting some helpful practices as much as we could benefit from living behind some distractive traditions. It is therefore crucial that we pay attention to our attitudes towards our bodies, how we treat our bodies, and the food we put in our bodies while we are in Diaspora. How we view and value these components will determine how we behave and who we are.

21

WE ARE WHAT WE EAT AND DO:

See to it that no one takes you captive by philosophy and empty deceit, according to human tradition, according to the elemental spirits of the world, and not according to Christ (Colossians 2:8).

A very powerful prayer line sermon enlightened me on who we are: We are Christian Zimbabweans in Diaspora. What was underscored during this sermon was that it is imperative that we identify ourselves first and foremost as Christians. Although this thinking might be taken for granted by some, for me this was an "Aha" moment. As Zimbabwean citizens, we have our valuable traditions in which we were raised and trained. Now living in Diaspora, we adopted new traditions. Historically both traditions have not stayed constant over the years, changing as the wind blows. Furthermore, not all practices are necessarily Biblically based. Christianity, on the other hand, has fixed traditions that are never changing and guarantee eternity. Well then, which traditions and lifestyles do we follow? One of the points that was being made in this sermon was that we need to know which Zimbabwean traditions to keep and which to throw away; which Diasporian practices to adopt and which not to adopt. The only way to help us decipher this dilemma is to use Biblical principles, thereby making us primarily Christian citizens.

The Lord knows that when two different worlds connect, one is more likely to take over. That is why He warns us against being enslavement by human and worldly traditions, but urges us to be Christ-led. Yes, it is possible to combine the two worlds together as long as they are compatible and one is able to select only those things that bring eternal life, and not have a life that is meaningless or not lasting. The choices we make should include selecting the right types of food considering what is available to us in Diaspora. For instance, we should try to obtain and eat naturally produced food. We should also be able to decide when and with whom we choose to share our food and how much we should eat. In addition, we should also maintain an active lifestyle, being aware of our daily physical activities or lack thereof.

Life in Diaspora has changed what we put on our tables; that is, if we still use the table for meal times at all. It has also changed how we get our food, prepare and store it. Furthermore, some of us have also changed our whole lifestyles and attitudes about the value of our bodies and the food we eat.

Technology and TV have replaced *pada*, and by default, we seem to have adopted a more sedentary lifestyle. Because of the two worlds that exist around us, we live challenging lives that require us to continually evaluate what we put on our plates and the types of lifestyles in which we participate. Knowing what we should eat and do is not enough as this environment continues to test us on how we should maintain what we know and believe. Our attitudes are the basis for how we welcome and react to these challenges.

WE ARE WHAT WE EAT AND DO:

So how do we respond to these changes and their effects on our health? We should ask ourselves the following questions:

What's on our plates?

What are our views of ourselves and the food we put in our body?

What we do on a day-to-day basis affects our health. The answer begins and ends with the Bible and us in between.

What I now know

In this chapter what I found most interesting is:

_____

_____

_____

_____

_____

~~~~

From this chapter I intend to do the following toward healthier eating:

_____

_____

_____

_____

_____

CHAPTER FOUR

ACTS: ZVIITO

I can do all things through him who strengthens me
(Philippians 4:13)

When we consider who we are, how we feel, and how we look, we cannot overlook contributions our actions or acts (*zviito zvedu*) have on our health. Our health is majorly dependent on how we choose to act. Yes, we can even say our genetics or our family medical history comes into play affecting how healthy we are. However, let us give thanks to our loving God who despite that provides encouragement all the time when our earthly eyes don't seem to find a way out, for the living Word says:

No, in all these things we are more than conquerors
through him who loved us (Romans 8:37).

Yes! God emphasizes In ALL THINGS, not SOME things! We are conquerors over anything and everything that is on and in our body, for who that is in us and loves us always makes make a way. As Believers, we know that being Christians does not mean that we do not suffer. Sometimes God makes a way for us around the situation while at times we have to go through it. Either way he goes with us and we have an option to stay with Him. First, we should believe that in spite of all, God has a specific and amazing individualized plan for each one of us. He promises to guide us and supply all our needs:

> *The LORD will guide you always; he will satisfy your*
> *needs in a sun-scorched land and will strengthen your*
> *frame. You will be like a well-watered garden, like a*
> *spring whose waters never fail (Isaiah 58:11).*

Therefore, with this assurance in mind, we should in any and all circumstances be encouraged to do the best we can to stay strong and healthy just like the well-watered garden and the spring whose water supply never fails. We need to focus on the nutrition that can foster healthy living and act in a manner that will help our bodies ward off sicknesses. When we talk about healthy lives, most of us start picturing our weakness and temptations on certain foods or behaviors. Nevertheless, let us remember that if we are ready and willing to take action (*kuita mabasa*), God is our pillar:

> *No temptation has overtaken you except what is common*
> *to mankind. And God is faithful; he will not let you be*
> *tempted beyond what you can bear. But when you are*
> *tempted, he will also provide a way out so that you*
> *can endure it (1Corinthians10:13)*

27

WE ARE WHAT WE EAT AND DO:

We cannot get rid of potential health hazards and risk factors by not doing anything. In addition to facing our responsibilities, having the types of foods that God provided for us, He also gave us a sound mind. We are then able to choose the right nutrition, have a capable body to act appropriately, and the Holy Spirit to lead us. All of the acts, *zviito*, start with having faith. Once we have faith, then our foundation for our acts, *(zviito zvedu)* will be solid.

> *Thus also faith by itself, if it does not have works, is dead*
> *(James 2:17).*

While our actions are based on our beliefs and faith, we should also honor and worship our God and His commands; He promises us health and long life:

> *Worship the Lord your God, and his blessing will be on*
> *your food and water. I will take away sickness from*
> *among you and none will miscarry or be barren in your*
> *land I will give you a full life span (Exodus 23:25-26).*

The promise for healthy long life here is very clear. God should be first in our lives. He should be worshipped before anything else, including food and our bodies. Yes, it is possible to love food and/or our bodies more than The Lord. This can be illustrated by how we can sometimes focus too much on how our bodies look to the point that we do not spent time with God. We can spend more time entertaining earthily things that gratify our bodies instead of spending time with God. We at times can disobey God by overeating or eating foods that we have been warned against and that have been proven by today's health scientists to cause illnesses. When we put our focus on the Lord, He promises us that everything else will fall into place, including disease and illness free bodies.

What I now know

In this chapter what I found most interesting is:

_____

_____

_____

_____

_____

~~~~

From this chapter I intend to do the following toward healthier eating:

_____

_____

_____

_____

_____

CHAPTER FIVE

HOW WE TAKE CARE OF OUR BODIES MATTERS

Do you not know that your bodies are temples of the
Holy Spirit, who is in you, whom you have received
from God? You are not your own; you were bought
at a price. Therefore honor God with your bodies
(1 Corinthians 6:19-20).

How many times have we heard that the Bible says that our body is a Temple? How many of us have actually stopped to think about what this means in terms of the food we put in our bodies-the Temple and our behaviors towards this Temple? How healthy we stay stems from the way we think of and treat our body. We are made of flesh in which God breathed His Spirit; therefore, our body, is a Temple in which the Holy Spirit dwells. If that is the case, why do some of us treat our body as if it is a garbage can? Why do we dump things in our body-The Temple, that are not healthy and have been proven since the beginning of time to be harmful? Why do we not keep our body, The Temple, clean and free from preventable diseases? Why do we let our body, The Temple, just sit there and not be active enough to stay healthy and therefore live a promised long life?

WE ARE WHAT WE EAT AND DO:

We have a sound mind and a capable body to do and make healthy decisions and healthy acts. On Sunday mornings, do we wake up and drag ourselves to church looking scruffy? No! We wake up, wash, and dress up in our Sunday best because we know we want to be presentable in church, the Temple of God that we keep clean and presentable. We also spiritually prepare our hearts for worship to receive the Word of God as we enter the church-Temple of God in order to keep our Spirit healthy. So if God says our body is The Temple, He means that we should keep it as clean as the church. Why then do we put foods inside our bodies that do not keep our inside clean and presentable as the church? These inquiries might sound harsh; however, God is not happy when we cover up our unhealthy eating and behaviors, for He sees all. We have to shine inside out! He wants us to be healthy in *ALL* things and not in *SOME* and that is why the Word says:

> *My loved one, it is my prayer that you may do well in all things and be healthy in body, even as your soul does well (3 John 1:2).*

The plan is simple: we should trust in the Lord and depend on His Word. It is therefore befitting that whatever we eat and do to our bodies should result in what is pleasing and presentable ONLY to God, not to this world, to our husbands and wives, or even to ourselves:

32

HOW WE TAKE CARE OF OUR BODIES MATTERS

Therefore, by the mercies of God, let us present our bodies
as a living sacrifice, holy and acceptable to God, which
is our spiritual worship (Romans 12:1).

This could be an "aha" moment that changes some of our minds and attitude toward a healthier living, using Biblical principles. Not everything that is done by the multitude is Biblical or pleasing to God. Just because we are in Diaspora, it doesn't mean that we should do as the local citizens do. The statement "When in Rome, do as the Romans do" does not mean we should follow all the nutrition and lifestyle of where ever we are, or that we should fit in the Diasporian way. The foundation of this phrase was from a 4th century Arch-bishop of Milan St. Ambrose, who wanted to minimize conflict over minor church traditions that were not grounded on any substantial problem. Therefore, to think that the origin of the statement was to encourage people to follow all the practices of the local people for the sake of wanting to blend in would be misrepresenting its intent. Therefore, not everything in Diaspora is substantial to healthy Christian living. That is why that which does not specifically go against the will of God should be easily dismissed. That is why the Arch-bishop's point about minor traditions versus substantial problems teaches us to focus on what is important, and not to "sweat the small stuff."

Back home, food was acquired, prepared, and eaten in certain ways that most of us now do not have the luxury to practice while in Diaspora. Reasons such as limited time, availability of ingredients and not having help come into play. That is why with the limited time we have, it is important to learn healthy eating methods using available ingredients. We have to focus on making our body an offering to God that is pleasing to His sight. As we adapt to ways of the new world trying to integrate our ways from the world we left behind, let us be vigilant and pray for the spirit of discernment to do the right thing and not just follow the world for the Word says:

> *Do not conform any longer to the pattern of this world,*
> *but be transformed by the renewing of your mind. Then*
> *you will be able to test and approve what God's will*
> *is-his good, pleasing and perfect will (Romans 12:2).*

Healthy living by eating nutritious food is not the only practice that contributes to presentable bodies. We need to be active. Yes, we need to get up and exercise. Our bodies were not created to be immobile. Having active lifestyles helps keep our bodies in shape and healthy. In the Bible, one of the characteristics of the virtuous woman of Proverbs 31 is described as having strength, which means she must be doing something active to keep her arms strong and firm:

> *She girds herself with strength and makes her*
> *arms strong and firm (Proverbs 31:17).*

This healthy woman does not get this quality by being idle and lazy which, by the way, God abhors. With a sense of humor, He lets us know:

> *But you, lazybones, how long will you sleep? When will*
> *you wake up? A little extra sleep, a little more slumber,*
> *a little folding of the hands to rest (Proverbs 6:9-10).*

I wonder if He is referring to some of us who have the habit of letting the alarm snooze three times every morning so we can get a little more slumber. The bottom line is that God is telling us that there is no room for laziness in a Christian's life. Our blessings and healthy living will not come from staying stagnant. Even scientist Newton's first law of motion states that an object in motion tends to remain in motion, and an object at rest tends to remain at rest. To be strong one has to be active, and to continue being active, one has to be strong.

What I now know

In this chapter what I found most interesting is:

_____

_____

_____

_____

_____

~~~~

From this chapter I intend to do the following toward healthier eating:

_____

_____

_____

_____

_____

CHAPTER SIX

HOW AND WHERE WE GET OUR FOOD MATTERS

These are the LORD's instructions: Each household
should gather as much as it needs. Pick up two
quarts for each person in your tent (Exodus 16:16).

As previously stated, long gone are the days when we used to go outside to pluck off green leafy vegetables of rape or *kovho*, tomatoes, and onions from our garden to be cooked for a meal on demand. Long gone also are the days of stone ground corn meal. These days we buy vegetables from the store with no knowledge of how they were produced, when they were plucked from their mother plant and how far they have travelled to get to our local stores. Today some of us prefer *ngwerewere*, a white as snow type of corn meal, rather than *mugaiwa*, a stone ground meal. In addition, some of us complain of how long it takes to cook *chi roadrunner* (natural raised chicken) because of its toughness.

Here in Diaspora, the mass production of fruits and vegetables calls for them to be picked and shipped well before the natural ripening process is completed. This is done mostly to minimize damage to the product so they can arrive in grocery stores looking colorful and fresh. However, when they are plucked from the tree or plant, they continue to grow without being fed from the mother plant and therefore do not get all the full natural nutrients not to mention that they are also sprayed with preservatives to lengthen their lifespan en route or on the shelf. Therefore, what we see is not usually what we get. This adds a completely new insight to healthy eating. Once removed from the produce's normal sources of water and nutrients, water losses and development changes cannot be prevented. From the time we buy the produce to the time we consume them, some nutrients would have deteriorated. This means that by the time we eat or cook the fresh vegetables or fruits, they are not as nutritious as we think. For example, vitamin C one of the most degradable vitamins, loses its effectiveness over a short time. Therefore, fruits and vegetables with vitamin C and even juices may have no vitamin C left in them if not consumed in as little as a week of being picked from the tree or from the time the juice bottle is opened.

For produce such as grains that require processing for further use, the more processed the grains, the less fiber and fewer nutrients than their counter parts. It is a fact that *ngwerewere* is more processed by grinding and sieving to be more appealing to the eye and for easier and faster cooking than *mugaiwa*. For instance, processing whole-wheat grain into white flour reduces the contents of vitamins B and E, fiber, and minerals, including zinc and iron. The sad thing is that these food preferences are leading us to not having enough nutrients in our food, which in turn leads to unhealthy conditions and diseases.

Since we now know that once picked vegetables and fruits immediately start to lose their nutritious value, it should matter to us how and where we get our food. If able, we should grow our produce. However, given that not many of us cannot keep a garden with fresh fruits and vegetables for use as needed, the best way to get nutrition is to buy fresh and from our local farmers. Buying directly from our local farmers, cuts down on the shipping and storage time, thereby keeping more of the produce nutrients intact. Furthermore, local grown produce is more likely to have less, if any, exposure to pesticides and contaminants. In addition, it is usually cheaper to buy from our local farmers than from organic stores. If there are not any local farmers available in the area, we can buy frozen produce with no additives as they are more nutrient-filled than some fresh bought produce. This is because frozen produce is plucked from its mother plant when it is fully developed and frozen right away, after blanching, to slow down deterioration, with no transport and storage time. Blanching is the process of dipping vegetables into boiling water, then removed after a short time, and then dipped into ice water or placed under cold running water to stop the cooking process while locking in freshness and flavor.

At times when we buy fresh produce, what we might think to be fresh might be at least a few weeks old and stripped of nutrients from the time it is plucked, transported, put on the store shelf, and then bought by us and stored on our counter tops or fridge. According to the Institute of Food Research, during this time produce like fresh beans can lose up to 45% of nutrients, broccoli and cauliflower 25%, garden peas up to 15%, and carrots up to 10%. Meanwhile, frozen peas contained up to 30% more vitamin C than fresh, and green beans up to 45% more.

That being said, some produce such as green leafy vegetables is even healthier eaten young than older. In this case, buying young is our best option nutrition wise. The leaves from baby green leafy vegetables such as spinach, kale, mustard greens and collards have been found to be more naturally active, meaning they have more nutrient value than older ones.

This brings us to the importance of how we acquire the food from the store because the way the food is displayed in the store makes a difference. Light has great influence on our food nutritious status, depending on the type of food. For instance, when we buy extra virgin olive oil, we want to make sure that it is not exposed to light as light depreciates the oil's nutritious value. Therefore, we should pick one that is in a tin can or reach way back on the shelf for a glass or plastic bottle that has not been exposed to too much light. On the other hand when picking up vegetables such as mushrooms or green vegetables, those that are more exposed to light have more nutrients such as vitamin and minerals.

With regards to the animal foods we eat, there is also need for concern on where they come from. We should all be aware that there are high levels of chemicals from industries, parasites, bacteria, and toxic wastes found in the waters that our seafood and so called fresh water fish come from. Some chemicals attach to animals such as fish and stay in the body. When we eat these fish, those chemicals can cause health issues as well as cause birth defects. Back home, we ate freshly fished *makwaya* (bream/tilapia) or *muramba* (catfish) from our local waters or Kariba dam. Today in the Diaspora we have no idea where most of the fish we eat comes from. Because of mass production farm fishing, the practice of raising fish commercially in tanks is a common and acceptable practice. Farmed fish are usually fed processed food, treated with antibiotics and are at risk for contamination. We should know where and how our fish is caught.

The way that the land animals we eat such as chicken and beef are raised also causes major concerns. Back home our cows and chicken were free roaming and naturally fed with grass for cows or natural grain for chicken. Chickens are meant to be free to scratch for insects, enjoy sunbaths, and roost in comfort. Cattle, goats, and lambs are truly contented as they graze on green pasture, breathe fresh air, and chew the cud as they stay on the farm from birth until they are slaughtered. Unless we breed our own chickens and cows or buy from our local farmers, the chicken meat and beef we buy in the regular grocery freezers are more likely bred for mass consumption. This means that they are likely to have been injected with antibiotics and hormones to improve their health, speed up their growth, and increase food production.

WE ARE WHAT WE EAT AND DO:

What these animals eat or are injected with is what is on our plates and is going into our bodies. Furthermore, these animals are also raised in confined places where there is not much room for movement. This results in unhealthy conditions for the animals, which causes them to be sick, and in turn, be treated with antibiotics. Some of these antibiotics may cause resistance when we are treated for infections. Since the animals are not free to roam around they don't develop strong healthy muscle meat and work off the fat to develop healthy lean fat.

Besides the obvious better tasting and texture of free-range, grass-fed, cud-chewing mammals, and natural grain fed pastured poultry, there are health benefits. Natural raised animal meat has more healthy protein, omega-3 fatty acids, and antioxidants. For egg lovers, no more throwing egg yolks away to lessen cholesterol on your plate. Farm raised eggs have:

- 1/3 less cholesterol
- 1/4 less saturated fat
- 2/3 more vitamin A
- 2 times more omega-3 fatty acids
- 3 times more vitamin E
- 7 times more beta carotene

Not only do we have to worry about how our animals and produce are raised, we also have to know if they are natural at all. Of late, there has been a lot of talk about GMOs. What are GMOs? GMO stands for Genetically Modified Organisms. They are plants or animals that have been genetically engineered, changed or modified with DNA from bacteria, viruses or other plants and animals. The reasons why GMOs exist are:

- Reduced need for herbicides
- Reduced need of pesticides
- Reduced greenhouse emissions as GMOs require less tillage or plowing, thus less use of fossil fuels
- Ability to manipulate foods to increase desirable components such as nutrients
- Increased production of food for starving third world countries.

As honorable as these reasons may be, one could still argue against all of them. The products of this process are unnatural. This production method may cause significant changes to these plants and animals, possibly producing undesirable effects on consumers. Our main concern is whether products made from this scientific approach are healthy for us to eat. There is a possibility that because of the way GMOs are produced, their unnatural structures may cause human organ damage, gastrointestinal and immune system disorders, accelerated aging, and infertility. It is also thought that if we eat any genetically modified food, they might leave some of the modified DNA inside us, which might possibly cause long-term health problems. The DNA genes inserted into genetically modified soy, for example, could possibly transfer into the DNA of bacteria living inside us. This is scary!

WE ARE WHAT WE EAT AND DO:

The way we can tell how food is genetically modified is usually by comparing it to its natural state. For example, we know that grapes, watermelon, or tomatoes were not created seedless. Therefore, as much as we love to gulp a mouthful of grapes or slice of watermelon without being disrupted to spit out the seeds, these forms of produce are not natural. The most genetically produced foods are corn because it feeds both humans and animals and soy as well, because it is the most versatile high protein and lean fat product. Some less obvious products are zucchini and squash, rice, wheat, potatoes, milk, and even salmon. As added ingredients to our foods, products such as sweetener-aspartame, vitamins, artificial and natural flavors are also found in genetically modified forms.

What I now know

In this chapter what I found most interesting is:

_____

_____

_____

_____

_____

~~~~

From this chapter I intend to do the following toward healthier eating:

_____

_____

_____

_____

_____

CHAPTER SEVEN

HOW WE PREPARE AND COOK OUR FOOD MATTERS

So Abraham hurried into the tent to Sarah, and said,
"Quickly, prepare three measures of fine flour, knead it
and make bread cakes. "Abraham also ran to the herd, and
took a tender and choice calf and gave it to the servant,
and he hurried to prepare it (Genesis 18:6-7).

Food practices such as selecting and paying attention to the type of food, how it is prepared, and cooking have been observed since the beginning of time. This is so important to us not only to our sense of smell and our taste buds but also because some nutrients are affected during this process.

Food preparation starts from the time we obtain the food, handle it and bring it in the house to when we cook it. There are many pollutants in the air, water, and environment that contaminate the crops and move through the food chain all the way to the food we eat. Care in selecting, preparation and cooking of our foods reduces the amounts of these contaminants consumed. We should therefore select a wide variety of foods to avoid excessive consumption of contaminants that may be present in any one food. Some of these impurities have been shown to possibly have negative effects on fetal and infant nervous systems, learning development, kidney health, brain development, and the risk of cancer.

We should be aware that most foods need thorough cleansing before cooking. In mass farming, pesticides are used to prevent diseases and insect invasion. Therefore, the fresh fruits and vegetables we buy in the stores require rinsing as they may have remnants of pesticides or even just to wash off soil, dirt, and fertilizer. Some of us have seen different kind of fruits and vegetable cleaners sold in the produce sections costing a bit more than we are willing to pay. A quick recipe for produce wash that we can make at home and use is as follows:

- 2tbs vinegar (natural disinfectant)
- 1cup water
- 1/2 lemon (for nice scent and also a natural disinfectant)
- *Option 1*(best for large produce like apples)

Pour in spray bottle and squeeze lemon (to make larger quantity, double or triple amounts)

Spray on produce rub and rinse for about 30 seconds

Option 2 (best for leafy vegetables or smaller fruits like berries)

Pour mixture in a bowl and soak produce for 2 minutes.

Rub and rinse for 30 seconds

WE ARE WHAT WE EAT AND DO:

We should also be aware of when and how to wash our produce. For the vegetables that are not cooked right away, it is best to wash, chop, and freeze them immediately until they are ready to be eaten. Just washing and storing them without freezing them in time speeds up ripening, which in turn results in rapid spoilage and mold formation. Ideally it is better not to buy produce in large amounts but to buy what we are going to use, since storing usually results in nutrient loss. As we chop and cut our different foods, it is recommended that we dedicate our cutting boards to either produce or meats to avoid cross contamination. In addition, using glass, plastic or bamboo cutting boards instead of wooden ones is advised to avoid harboring of bacteria in the cracks on wooden boards.

We also have to think twice about cooking. There are several ways to cook our food, namely boiling, baking, steaming, frying, broiling, barbequing/*braaing,* or roasting. How we choose to cook can determine the type of nutrients we lose and provide for ourselves. Some types of cooking can destroy some nutrients such as antioxidants. Boiling makes it easier for nutrients to leak into the water and be lost when drained, unless we intend to drink the nutrients in that water as soup. Over-cooking using any method also diminishes nutrients by breaking down their food cells. It is then advised to use as little water as possible when cooking vegetables. Usually the water left in the vegetables from washing or in frozen vegetables is enough to steam the vegetables without boiling them. Other types of cooking such as frying can add ingredients that we do not need like trans-fat or cholesterol. Both approaches of cooking can lead to bad health by either destruction of nutrients or addition of unhealthy ingredients.

Temperature can also affect the food we cook. Using high-temperature methods, such as pan frying or grilling directly over an open flame for a long period, is not recommended. Though there are still studies in progress, the National Cancer Institute (NCI) states that chemicals are formed when meat, including beef, pork, fish, and poultry, is cooked using high-temperature methods, such as pan frying or grilling directly over an open flame. These chemicals have been found to cause changes in DNA that may increase the risk of cancer. The NCI also suggests the following cooking practices to reduce the production of these chemicals:

- Avoid direct exposure of meat to an open flame or a hot metal surface
- Avoid prolonged cooking times (especially at high temperatures)
- Continuously turn meat over on a high heat source instead of leaving the meat on the heat source for a while without flipping over
- Cut off charred portions of meat
- Refraining from using gravy made from meat drippings

Overall, nutrients can be preserved when there is less contact with water, shorter cooking times, and less exposure to heat. Therefore, to preserve nutrients, methods such as steaming, stir-frying, sautéing, using a tight-fitting lid when possible, and baking at the right temperature without added fat, are recommended just as baking was for Elijah years ago:

> He looked around, and there by his head was some bread baked over hot coals, and a jar of water. He ate and drank and then lay down again (1 Kings 19:16).

To further preserve more nutrients, cooking fruits and vegetables as a whole or without peeling their skins on is advisable. For instance, the following foods are best eaten with their skin: sweet potatoes, cucumbers, squash, and citrus fruits. Yes, citrus peels are rich in antioxidants and bad cholesterol lowering flavonoids. Citrus peels can be grated over vegetables or added to whole grain muffins. In addition, we should not throw away healthy celery leaves or broccoli stalks and leaves.

Some foods such as beans are better prepared for better cooking by soaking. Most people know that we soak beans to make them tender, thereby reducing cooking time. There are more good reasons why we should soak our beans before cooking. The first major reason that would be appreciated by most is that soaking beans minimizes gas. While beans are soaking, the indigestible complex sugars are removed from the outer coating of the beans. This results in reduction of bloating and gas. The next reason is as previously discussed that shorter cooking times preserved nutrients. Soaking beans cuts down the cooking time from possibly 2 hours to 15 minutes if cooked with a pressure cooker. Another reason is that as the beans soak, they slowly absorb the liquid they need to cook evenly and completely so they don't split open, lose their skins and nutrients, or cook only the outer surface while the middle remains hard. Finally, bean soaking also removes a lot of dirt from the bean skin, while it preserves the proteins, vitamins and minerals inside.

One of my favorite finger licking versatile bean dishes that takes me back home is *rupiza*. Back home, *nyemba* (cow peas) alone or with *nyimo* were used to make this dish. It is as versatile as it can be enjoyed with any main meal as a protein side with *sadza* as well as a dip with appetizers. My mom's family recipe modified to include a variety of legumes found here in Diaspora for a fine tasting *rupiza* is as follows:

- 1/4 cup black eyed peas
- 1/4 cup Pinto beans
- 1/4 black beans
- 1/4 cup lentils
- 1/4 cup split peas
- 1 cup peanut butter
- 1 large tomato
- 1 large onion
- Extra virgin olive oil
- Cayenne pepper to taste
- Salt to taste

WE ARE WHAT WE EAT AND DO:

- Soak black eyed peas, pinto beans, and black beans overnight or for at least 12 hours in water- make sure water is at least 2 inches over the beans.
- Drain all the water and let stand till dry
- Blend the dried beans a few at a time to small pieces
- Put all blended beans, lentils and split peas in a pressure cooker and cook for 30 minutes or in a regular pot till soft
- Add salt and cayenne pepper to taste
- In a separate pot, make an onion and tomato stew
- Add the well-cooked stew to the pot of beans and mix till all ingredients are blended smoothly together in a porridge consistency. Enjoy!

What I now know

In this chapter what I found most interesting is:

_____

_____

_____

_____

_____

~~~

From this chapter I intend to do the following toward healthier eating:

_____

_____

_____

_____

_____

CHAPTER EIGHT

HOW AND WHERE WE STORE OUR FOOD MATTERS

These are the Lord's instructions: "Each household should gather as much as it needs. Pick up two quarts for each person in your tent." So the people of Israel did as they were told. Some gathered a lot some only a little. But when they measured it out, everyone had just enough. Those who gathered a lot had nothing left over, and those who gathered only a little had enough. Each family had just what it needed. Then Moses told them, "Do not keep any of it until morning." But some of them didn't listen and kept some of it until morning. But by then it was full of maggots and had a terrible smell. Moses was very angry with them. After this the people gathered the food morning by morning, each family according to its need. And as the sun became hot, the flakes they had not picked up melted and disappeared (Exodus 16:16-21).

Why did God specifically instruct the Israelites only to gather enough food needed for the day and not to keep any leftovers? God could have just provided the food and let His children gather and eat as they pleased without any instructions at all. However, why was it so important that they gather as much as they needed not wanted? It is because a lesson on trust and dependence on God was being taught. When the Israelites were in the wilderness, God wanted to teach them to have faith in Him. He wanted them to rely and believe in Him. He also wanted to show them that He could provide for them even when it seemed impossible and that they should not have to worry about where food would come from going forth.

So how does this lesson apply to us today in our Diasporian wilderness? We now know that regularly buying fresh food in bulk is does not preserve nutrition. Besides our food losing the needed nourishment the longer we store it, we should, like the Israelites, also learn to trust God and try to buy just enough to cook for a few days and believe in God for tomorrow as He said:

> *Therefore do not worry about tomorrow, for tomorrow will worry about itself. Each day has enough trouble of its own (Mathew 6:34).*

In addition to us not getting the best benefits from the food we buy in bulk, sometime we end up wasting the food when we do not store it properly before and after it is cooked. How many of us have thrown away that brown/black bunch of bananas from the fruit basket? Even after we buy just enough to cook for a few days, what we do with leftovers matters. How many containers from the fridge have we opened and sniffed to see if the contents are still edible before we threw them away? When in the wilderness, in Diaspora, we cannot afford to waste a penny. In the above scenario, we are reminded that when the Israelites in the wilderness gathered more than they needed, it all decayed.

Is this book not supposed to offer practical suggestions? How practical is it for most of us to go grocery shopping every day in Diaspora. There are valid reasons why we do buy some things in bulk. Most of the time it is usually because the food is on sale or that we only have limited opportunity to go to the store. In any case, in the event that more is bought than can be consumed at the time, it is important that we know how to make sure we get the most and best out of our food, by using the best storage methods. Cold foods should be kept cold until they are served and frozen foods kept frozen and thawed in the refrigerator before cooking. Yes, when in doubt about the safety of a food, discard it.

Food storage includes that which is not cooked and left overs. When we buy more food than we can cook at the time, produce, for example, should be stored intact as a whole. Cutting up the fruits and vegetables and then leaving them out on the counter or storing them in open containers will cause 10-25% of antioxidants like vitamin C and carotenoids to dissipate over the course of a week, because of exposure to oxygen. Cutting up produce also exposes fruits and vegetable pores, thereby releasing compounds that speed up ripening and spoilage. When juicing fruits and vegetables, it is advised to juice and drink right away, as leaving the juice over several days will make it lose its nutrients.

For any vegetables that are not eaten immediately, specific methods can be used for different vegetables to effectively preserve them. For green, leafy vegetables, it is advised to cut them, blanch them as previously described then immediately freeze them in zip lock freezer bags. On the other hand, produce such as mushrooms can be left on the counter under the light for ultra-violet enhancement as discussed before.

When packing produce in the refrigerator or counter, it is best to pack loosely, separating each item by its type. The closer the fruits and vegetables are to each other, the faster they will ripen and rot. Therefore, it is advised to separate fruits in different drawers from surrounding vegetables, especially apples, as they can turn leafy greens and other veggies brown. Ties and rubber bands should be removed and produce stored loosely in perforated paper, plastic, or cloth wrapping in order not to suffocate the produce. Tomatoes are best stored on their own and not in plastic bags as they are likely to ripen more quickly. Tomatoes can also be blanched and stored frozen. Most vegetables are best stored in the crisper drawer at the bottom of the fridge. However, garlic, onions, potatoes, shallots, sweet potatoes, and winter squash can be stored in a cool and dark pantry. Note that potatoes and onions are only great together when they are cooked. Before that, they should not be stored next to each other, as they both will release moisture and gases that will cause the other to spoil faster. It is important to keep in mind that these storage recommendations are time limited unless frozen stored (See APPENDIX A for more ways to preserve food nutrients).

WE ARE WHAT WE EAT AND DO:

Another very healthy way to preserve food with a longer shelf life is dehydration. This process, known to make *mufushwa* (from dried vegetables) or *chimukuyu* (biltong from dried meat), dates back to good old Zimbabwe days when it was a necessity. Although using good old fashion methods of drying the food in the sun, today's modern technology provides dehydrators. Dehydration of food preserves almost all the nutrients. In addition to vegetables and meats, fruits can also enjoyed with a remarkable array of concentrated flavor and nutrients when dehydrated.

What I now know

In this chapter what I found most interesting is:

_____

_____

_____

_____

_____

~~~~

From this chapter I intend to do the following toward healthier eating:

_____

_____

_____

_____

_____

CHAPTER NINE

WHAT WE EAT AND HOW MUCH FOOD MATTERS

When you sit down to dine with a ruler, consider carefully what is before you, And put a knife to your throat if you are a man of great appetite (Proverbs 23:1-2).

When we finally sit down to eat is the moment that most of us fall prey to some unhealthy nutritious habits. Even after we have done everything from selecting healthy fresh and nutrition-filled foods, healthily preparing and storing the rest, to cooking our meals as recommended, the types and amount of food we eat is also concerning with regards to our health. We should seriously consider what is in front of us before we put it in our mouths.

There is no doubt that many factors affect what and how much we eat. To name a few, our financial status can influence the types of food we buy based on what we can afford and the price of the food. In addition, food availability is a big factor if we are trying to eat healthy and do not have access to the products we need. As discussed before, time is definitely a factor that controls what we eat. Sometimes we are constrained with our day to day hustle and bustle that we end up picking up fast food for our kids when we are tired and do not have time to cook. Most of our kids do not mind this at all; however, most fast foods are full of preservatives, are high in sugar and salt content, as well as being made from unhealthy processed ingredients.

It also does not help when everywhere we turn we see and hear on TV, radio and billboards, food commercials on the latest food invention offered for a limited time at a lower price. Furthermore, we also have our not so healthy habits and routines as well as life styles due to our busy schedules. For instance, some of us have adopted routine habits of driving by Starbucks and Krispy Kreme for a cup of coffee and doughnut every morning on our way to work. Some of us have introduced pizza night every Friday night as a fun family dinner. We also have some not so healthy traditions or customs of frying vegetables in a lot of oil or using a lot of salt in our cooking. While attending social events involving food and drinks is not necessarily a bad indulgence from time to time, we are encouraged to approach these occasions with caution. Knowledge is power and without it, we perish:

My people perish because of lack of knowledge (Hosea 4:6).

Having self-control is the foundation of how we can decide what we should eat and how much. Just because the food presented to us is healthy, it also does not mean that we should eat a lot or all of it. Even too much water is not good for us, and yes, there is such a thing as water intoxication. We also know that there is also such a thing as overeating. Moreover, there are consequences to every action including overindulgence on food. That is why God tells us not to let our appetite get the best of us.

> *"If you find honey, eat just enough–too much of it, and you will vomit" (Proverbs 25:16).*

If vomiting were the only bad consequence of overeating, it would not be so bad. However, we all know that we put ourselves at bad health risks when we overeat or eat unhealthily.

What then drives us to want to eat? Is it appetite or hunger? If it is one or both, is there a difference between appetite and hunger anyway? In fact, there is. Hunger is more of a biological or physiological drive. When we are hungry, it means that our body is lacking nutrients needed to make our bodies function. As nutrients are digested and absorbed by the stomach and small intestine, they are sent to needed parts for our body to use. Signals are then sent to the liver and brain messaging reduction of further food intake. In our wonderfully made body, God installed a thermostat called the hypothalamus. Although there are many factors that play into our satiety or being full, the hypothalamus helps regulate whether we should eat or not. The process starts with us eating the food and completes with actions in the hypothalamus telling us that we are full. Not only did God, our merciful Father wonderfully and efficiently create us with this thermostat, but He instilled chemicals for hunger and satiety in our body that help our bodies make the right decisions about when to eat and to stop. As much as we have the hunger hormone in the lining of our stomach that alerts us when we are hungry, we also have a hormone that tells our brain when we are full. Thus, this mechanism that was divinely installed in us is to keep our bodies alive without over-eating. It is for our survival.

Appetite, on the other hand, is psychologically driven. This system is affected by external food choices, such as seeing a tempting dessert or smelling cooked food. Emotionally triggered factors such as depression, anxiety, loneliness, boredom, and stress can urge us to want to eat comfort foods or overeat in order to fill that emotional void. What about cravings? A craving is an intense desire to eat something specific. Causes of cravings are still a subject of discussion. However, situations that cause chemical imbalances such as menstruation in women and stress in everyone, have been linked to cravings.

As much as we should enjoy eating our food, we are supposed to eat to live, not live to eat. As much as there are "see food diets" (I see it, I eat it), let us also remember: "out of sight, out of mind." This means that we do not have to eat everything we see and is pleasing to our eyes and nose, and if we keep away what we don't need and that which is not so healthy, we won't easily see it to reach out and eat it. Because we tend to eat more when we have easy access to food, we can make our homes health-friendly zones, by replacing candy dishes with fruit dishes and not displaying cookies and chips on our tables and counter tops. We could also practice self-control for portion control. When looking at our plate, the size of our meat serving (example chicken, fish, or beef) should be the size of our palm, not the whole hand. Our starches, example *sadza* rice or potatoes, should be the size of our round handful. It is very much encouraged to eat as much vegetables as we can even if the serving portion is more than that of the protein and starch. Finally, we should practice eating slowly so that our brain can get the message on time when our stomach is full.

Having the thermostat and hormones installed in us, do we always listen to our bodies, or do we let feelings like appetite, cravings, or dare we say glutton, take precedence? Glutton or overeating is the work of the flesh. The flesh wants what it wants or craves whenever and however it wants. We know that listening to the flesh can get us in trouble. The story of one brother who sold his birthright due to fleshly demands of hunger in the Bible is a perfect example. This brother was willing to give up his future and his inheritance because his flesh could only see today:

> *Once when Jacob was cooking some stew, Esau came*
> *in from the open country, famished. He said to Jacob,*
> *"Quick, let me have some of that red stew! I'm famished.*
> *Jacob replied, "First sell me your birthright." "Look, I am*
> *about to die," Esau said. "What good is the birthright to*
> *me? "But Jacob said, "Swear to me first." He swore an*
> *oath to him, selling his birthright to Jacob. Then Jacob*

gave Esau some bread and some lentil stew. He ate and
drank, and then got up and left (Genesis - 25:2934).

This is not a parable. It is a true story. For some of us, this might seem to have been the most ridiculous thing ever. Was Esau that hungry or was the meal that appetizing that he could not wait for dinner, to the point that he was willing to trade in his livelihood? At one point or the other, we have given up or risked something valuable to us for food due to desires of our flesh. We risk our health every time we put empty calories, fatty foods, or any unhealthy food in our mouths. These risks have potential for unhealthy conditions such as obesity, heart diseases, diabetes, stroke, chronic joint pains, cancer, and yes, even death. The greatest gift that Jesus left us with the Holy Spirit to help us when the flesh seems to overpower our will. We know that for He said:

"But I say, walk by the Spirit, and you will not carry out
he desire of the flesh. For the flesh sets its desire against
the Spirit, and the Spirit against the flesh for these are
in opposition to one another, so that you may not do the things
that you please" (Galatians 5:16).

As we consider what is on our plates, let us not allow our flesh and the Spirit to play tug of war with each other. Let us not believe what everyone or even what our body is telling us. Let's

WE ARE WHAT WE EAT AND DO:

believe the living Word. We can start by asking ourselves:

> "Do I need to eat THIS?" (type of food)
> "Do I need to eat ALL of this?" (amount of food?)
> "WHAT ELSE can I substitute in place of that?" (options of
> healthy foods).

By ourselves we cannot do it, but by having faith and with the help of the fruit of the Spirit of self-control, we can prevail:

> *But the fruit of the Spirit is love, joy, peace, patience,*
> *kindness goodness, faithfulness, gentleness, self-control;*
> *against such things there is no law (Galatians 5:22-23).*

When we have self-control, we are able to select the most important healthy foods over our needs, cravings, appetite and even hunger. These conditions can make room for us to grab whatever is in front of us to fill the immediate need. When we have self-control, we also have the wisdom to be governed by principle instead of feelings or appearances. Self-control is using our strength to choose God's will for us in order to be healthy and forsaking anything else that is competing with our Holy Spirit. Despite the discouragement or self-doubt the devil will whisper to us, we have the power to overcome:

> *For God gave us a spirit not of fear but of power and love*
> *and self-control (2Timothy 1:7).*

We have the ability to say "No" to anything in excess or anything unhealthy that should not go in our bodies and defile the Temple. We have the power over our appetites and mouths.

Therefore, we are not to let them control us, but guard them. So, as we consider what we are getting ready to eat, let us make sure that first of all our plates show a picture of health, and then direct our attention to our mouths:

> *Set a guard, O Lord, over my mouth; keep watch over the*
> *door of my lips! (Psalm 141:3).*

What I now know

In this chapter what I found most interesting is:

_____

_____

_____

_____

_____

~~~

From this chapter I intend to do the following toward healthier eating:

_____

_____

_____

_____

_____

CHAPTER TEN

WITH WHOM WE EAT OUR FOOD MATTERS

For where two or three are gathered in my name, there
am I among them" (Mathew 18:20).

Most of us can attest to how food, especially a menu that involves *sadza, nyama, nemuriwo* tends to taste better and is more enjoyable where two or more are gathered. This is called fellowshipping. When God made us, He did not want for us to be alone; therefore, He created families, relatives, and friends for our companionship. When we gather in His name, He promises to be there. Families are to live, celebrate, laugh, share, eat, and pray together. Yet as we get together to eat, we are advised to choose appropriate companionship and warned against dining with those with bad influence:

> *Do not be with heavy drinkers of wine, Or with*
> *gluttonous eaters of meat (Proverbs 23:20).*

We should however, not be ashamed to enjoy our blessing of the food provided by God. He wants us to take pleasure in

WE ARE WHAT WE EAT AND DO:

what we eat while we are on this earth. That is why He also gave us the strength to work on our land and produce food so we can sit back and enjoy the fruits of our labor:

> *Then I realized that it is good and proper for a man to eat and drink, and to find satisfaction in his toilsome labor under the sun during the few days of life God has given him--for this is his lot (Ecclesiastes 5:18).*

> *A person can do nothing better than to eat and drink and find satisfaction in their own toil. This too, I see, is from the hand of God (Ecclesiastes 2: 24).*

Being in Diaspora, finding time to sit together every day with our families can be a challenge. When we grew up back home, we looked forward to enjoying our family time together at home. Sometimes our working parents would even come home for lunch, and in the evening we would wait till everyone was home before sitting down to eat. This is as God intended as He gave us simple instructions to eat together and eat at home:

> *So then, my brothers, when you come together to eat, wait for each other. If anyone is hungry, he should eat at home… (1Corinthians 11:34a).*

Some of us might even recall the joy that filled our homes when we sat and ate with our parents while they told us funny stories. In the country family fellowshipping extended beyond dinnertime as all the neighboring kids joined us to gather around the fire and intensely pay attention to *ambuya* (grandmother) or *sekuru* (grandfather) relate a folktale:

"Paivapo" "Once upon a time", is how every tale started.
"Dzefunde" "Go on", we would eagerly respond.
"Tsuro na gudo..." "A baboon and a hare..." the story would
go on.
"...Ndopakaperera sarungano." "...This is where the story ends," is how each story was concluded.

We all enjoyed these narrations that were richly dressed with sing-a-long songs and drama; however their main purpose was to teach us life lessons, and in them came lessons such as not to be greedy, to be patient, to respect others, and to be thankful. Some would enjoy this moment feasting on a desert of *Mxanla* (sweet corn and pumpkin dish made as follows:

Proportions of ingredients are based on personal taste where some prefer more corm and other more *mashamba*.

- samp (corm/maize)
- *Mashamba* (butternut squash or pumpkin)
- Brown sugar

WE ARE WHAT WE EAT AND DO:

Cook samp till tender

Add chopped up *mashamba* and cook till tender

Add brown sugar to taste

Sikai (whisk) till *mashamba* are blended

Most enjoy this dish cold, but can be served hot

Given our situation in Diaspora, any opportunity to eat together as a family is encouraged even if it is that one day a week when everyone is home. Eating together as a family allows open communication and getting to know what is going on in each family member's life. Concerns and issues can be raised and discussed while listening to how everybody's day went.

> *Not neglecting to meet together, as is the habit of some,*
> *but encouraging one another… (Hebrews10:25a).*

Our environment in Diaspora today is different from the one most of us knew back home. Our children face so many challenges and pressures from their friends and the society around them. Teenage years are one of the toughest life milestones to get through. This is the time adolescents tend to think that they are invincible and therefore are more likely to experiment with anything and anyone. Letting our children talk and ask questions at the dinner table instills confidence and trust in them, making them feel valued. As experienced and caring adults, we can take this opportunity to show interest and ask our children about school, sports, friends, and daily activities. This is also time for us as parents to pay attention to the children's needs, talk about facts of life, encourage them to open up and teach them how to pray. It is then we might be able to foresee and prevent some negative consequences of today and tomorrow. Meal-times are also teachable moments when our children can learn about Christian life values. These can be done through story-telling, Bible principles or any format, as the Lord instructs:

> *Start children off on the way they should go, and even*
> *when they are old they will not turn from it (Proverbs*
> *22:6).*

In this day and era of high technology, the gadgets we all own can serve as distraction. To make family dinner time even more valuable, we should turn off the TV, music, and yes, cell phones. This way everyone can focus on each other and what is being said. When there is no interest in what is going on in the family, the whole family unit can fall apart. Every part of the member needs to work together and support each other. Whatever the discussions at the table, it should be to build each other up, for the Bible says:

> *Two are better than one, because they have a good reward for*
> *their toil. For if they fall, one will lift up his fellow. But woe*
> *to him who is alone when he falls and has not another to lift*

him up! Again, if two lie together, they keep warm, but how can one keep warm alone? And though a man might prevail against one who is alone, two will withstand him a threefold cord is not quickly broken (Ecclesiastes 4:9-12).

Oh yes, there are some of us who like to eat out. There is absolutely nothing wrong with that as long as we do not neglect our homes. Dining at home is preferred more often that eating out as we tend to eat healthier at home than in restaurants. Although many restaurants have added calorie labels on their menus, we don't ever know all the ingredients and additives that are put in our meals. Furthermore, because restaurants tend to serve more than recommended healthy portions, some of us end up eating more than what we would have eaten at home. When eating out, one good practice is to request a to-go box before eating in order to split the serving into healthy portions.

What I now know

In this chapter what I found most interesting is:

_____

_____

_____

_____

_____

~~~~

From this chapter I intend to do the following toward healthier eating:

_____

_____

_____

_____

_____

CHAPTER ELEVEN

WHEN WE EAT OR DON'T EAT OUR FOOD MATTERS

And you shall eat and be full, and you shall bless the lord your God for the good land he has given you (Deuteronomy 8:10).

Are there specific times or situations that we are supposed to eat or not eat? The Word says when we eat we shall be full, which means that we should be able to limit ourselves to eating until we are full when we are hungry. We are also told to feed our enemies and strangers when they are hungry:

If your enemy is hungry, give him food to eat; if he is thirsty, give him water to drink (Proverbs 25:21).

We should also be able to stop eating when we are satisfied, not when all the food on our plate is gone! Some of us might still hear a voice from the past telling us not to leave the table until all the food on our plate is gone. Though this might have been said due to our parents not wanting to waste food after working so hard to get it on the table, this might have inadvertently instilled unhealthy behaviors that today make us feel like we have to finish what is on our plates. If that is a familiar experience for any of us, today we should strive to deprogram that voice from trying to empty the plate to eating only until we are full or satisfied. The Bible says Jesus fed multitudes when they were hungry till they were satisfied, not till all the food was gone:

> *They all ate and were satisfied, and the disciples picked up twelve basketfuls of broken pieces that were left over (Mathew 14: 20).*

When Israelites were hungry in the wilderness, God provided food for them so they would not go hungry. So was the case with Elijah when he was hungry. We should try not eating when our body deceives us by tempting us toward unhealthy desires or telling us we are craving certain foods. That is when we tend to overeat and eat unhealthy foods.

With regards to when we should eat and not eat, the Bible does not appear to have specific guidance, whether it should be three square meals that we grew up accustomed to or several small meals recommended by today's dieticians. In the case mentioned above, Elijah was fed by the raven that brought him food in the morning and in the evening. What we learn the most in the Bible about food is not to overeat, and that certain foods are healthy while others are not. We also learn that we should trust in the Lord to provide food for us daily:

Give us this day our daily bread (Mathew 6:11).

As Christians, there are times when some of us give up food when we fast. There are other times when some of us also give up food when we diet. These two important topics will be discussed separately in the following chapters as they need more attention. What we can address here with regards to when we should or should not eat is the significance of skipping meals and its connection to our health.

There is a theory that skipping meals can result in gaining weight. The concept behind this is that when we skip meals or eat one meal a day, our body thinks that it is starving and therefore holds on to whatever is available as future energy reserve. It stores this energy in the form of fat. In the event that the body actually starves, the body can then go to the "reserve tank" of fat which would be converted to energy. However, we know that, for instance normally if we eat dinner as our only meal of the day, our next dinner time will soon come and the stored fat will not get used up. Because we don't get to starve, the stored fat then settles nicely around our belly, causing weight gain. Keeping this in mind, it should be highlighted that skipping a few meals would not trigger the body into this starvation mode of weight gain. If behavior is continued, however, the starvation mode will be triggered. Therefore, skipping meals throughout the day in favor of eating only one meal per day is not a quick ticket to losing weight, under the assumption that we are eating fewer calories. Yes, first the weight loss might occur as the body would not immediately realize what is going on, and if the behavior continues, the body will go into the protective storage mode.

What about breakfast being the most important meal of the day, and what about not eating after 6 pm? How does this all fit in with when we should eat in order to stay healthy; and most of all, gaining or losing weight?

There is an ongoing debate on whether skipping breakfast is healthy or even whether eating in bed will make us gain weight. Reviewed literature, together with personal experience, and a healthcare practitioner, suggests good news for everyone. Apparently, both skipping breakfast and eating breakfast within two hours of waking up as recommended can produce good health benefits. Studies show that NOT skipping breakfast is associated with:

- decreased overall appetite
- decreased overall food consumption
- decreased body weight
- improved academic performance
- improved blood sugar control

Skipping breakfast on the other end is associated with:

- increased fat breakdown

- increased release of growth hormone (which has anti-aging and fat loss benefits)
- improved blood glucose control
- improved cardiovascular function
- decreased food intake

To get an understanding of how this could be working, let us explore the recommendations that come with when we should be eating. Here is a commonly recommended healthy eating schedule that is said to boost our metabolism:

- 6-8 a.m.: Breakfast
- 10 a.m.: Snack
- 12-2 p.m.: Lunch
- 3-4 p.m.: Snack
- 5-6 p.m.: Dinner
- 7-p.m.: Snack
- Don't eat after 7 p.m.

Then what is metabolism anyway? Metabolism is basically how our bodies process chemicals to keep us alive. How is it linked to weight gain and weight loss? Is it not said that the more we process or use chemicals like calories, the less we store and therefore the less weight we gain? As it turns out, metabolism state is a genetic disposition we have in our bodies; which some people are blessed to be born having high metabolism. People who have high metabolism are the ones we see eating anything and everything while packing desserts down, and not gain an ounce of weight. And yet there are those who, no matter what they nibble on or put on their celery, they have to be carefully not to tip the scale over. Yes, it is not fair, but thank God for the One and only Who is in us, Who created a gateway to boost our metabolism. For those not predisposed with the gene of high metabolism, there are ways of improving this system.

Let us now consider the person who follows the six small meals a day regiment. It would make sense that most people who tend to follow this kind of proposed plan will also tend to eat the healthy recommended foods at the given times. It also adds up that it is very unlikely that this person's breakfast will include chocolate doughnuts with a whole milk latte and an omelet, a burger for lunch, and spaghetti with garlic bread for dinner while snacking on snickers bars or even a banana at their best. Most of the time the meals and snacks recommended when eating small meals are as follows:

- **Breakfast** - Egg, slice of whole-wheat toast, and half a grapefruit
- **Snack** - An apple with a piece of cheese and light popcorn
- **Lunch** - Waldorf salad and half a turkey sandwich
- **Snack** - Smoothie made with yogurt, fruit, and juice
- **Dinner** - Grilled chicken sandwich with veggies

WE ARE WHAT WE EAT AND DO:

It is obvious that the types of food that are recommended are healthy. What is more important are the benefits and role these foods play individually and in combination, with the idea of eating several times a day. What exactly is going on when we follow these recommendations of eating breakfast early, eating several meals throughout the day and not eating late? For instance based on the example of suggested food types:

- They have high fiber and protein content- make us feel fuller.
- Several meals a day help to curb our cravings
- Several meals a day keep us satiated- full, leaving no room for hunger
- Small meals several times a day decrease binge eating and gorging
- Right portions of carbohydrates, protein, and fat can lower glycemic index and keep blood sugar stable
- Several meals a day encourage more fat burning while in the "fed" instead of "starvation" state all day long
- Right types of food offer less calories

Okay, so we can now address the burning questions about eating within two hours of waking up to speed up metabolism, whether to skip or not to skip breakfast, and whether to eat late. Then, does it really matter when we should eat or not eat our food? Yes and no. It does matter depending on medical conditions we might have. There are certain times when it is healthier than others to eat our meals. However, with regards to weight gain and weight loss, it actually does not matter when we eat our food. It is more important how much and what we eat during the day. Calories in, calories out should be our mantra. If we eat more calories than we use up, even if they are coming from healthy foods, we will gain weight no matter what time of the day we are eating. Any excess calories will turn into fat. The answer to the leading inquiries then is that we should relax and do what fits our life styles, as long as what ultimately goes in our mouth is healthy, balanced, and proportional and what goes out in a form of physical activity is more or same in calorie amounts we consume.

In general, however, skipping meals, does not give our body the steady energy supply we need to properly function throughout the day. In addition, skipping meals allows us to reach that hunger level where we tend to consume just about any first thing we see and forget when to stop. The theory of starvation may also apply if we make it a habit of going too long without eating. Most of all it is important to keep in mind that skipping meals is not a healthy way to diet. Aside from the time we set aside to fast, skipping meals as a regular practice is not advised, and we should at all times eat regularly and healthily.

What I now know

In this chapter what I found most interesting is:

_____

_____

_____

_____

_____

~~~~

From this chapter I intend to do the following toward healthier eating:

_____

_____

_____

_____

_____

CHAPTER TWELVE

FASTING

There is a time for everything, and a season for every activity under heaven (Ecclesiastes 3:1).

As Christians, we know that there is certainly time to eat and time to give up food, temporarily. Just like battery operated gadgets that need recharging, we need to get our Spirit recharged constantly to stay rejuvenated in the Word. There is power in fasting. It can be done individually or corporately. Esther knew that. When she was faced with a reality of a whole nation going to perish, she chose to tap into God's power to overcome evil using corporate fasting. Fasting gave her strength and confidence to face the king and do the unthinkable.

Then Esther told them to reply to Mordecai, "Go, gather all the Jews to be found in Susa, and hold a fast on my behalf, and do not eat or drink for three days, night or day. I and my young women will also fast as you do. Then I will go to the king, though it is against the law, and if I perish, I perish" (Esther 4:15-16).

WE ARE WHAT WE EAT AND DO:

What is fasting and why should Christians participate in fasting? In general, fasting is giving up food for a limited time while focusing on the living Word and prayer. It is a spiritual discipline. Fasting is time spent with God instead of food. It is a fact that when we fast, we are likely to feel hunger pains. We are encouraged to use those moments as reminders that we are hungry in order to get to know our Lord Jesus, and that we rely on Him for every need. We should then pray and ask the Holy Spirit to give us strength, lead us not into temptation for food, and deepen our understanding and experience of Jesus in our everyday life. Although we can read the Word and pray every day, adding a fast to the mix, helps us focus on what is important and makes us hunger more for God. When we fast we choose to sacrifice food in exchange for a relationship with God.

People fast for different reasons. Most of us fast when times are tough and we need a miracle or need to see major changes in our lives. That is okay. That is what Jesus meant when he told the disciples:

"This kind can come out by nothing but prayer and fasting"
(Mark 9:29).

At other times we fast to seek guidance and direction just as Paul and Barnabas did as they were appointing elders in the church:

> *Paul and Barnabas appointed elders for them in each church*
> *and, with prayer and fasting, committed them to the Lord,*
> *in whom they had put their trust (Acts 14:23).*

Other times we fast because we need to overcome temptation just like our Lord Jesus. When Jesus fasted for 40 days and nights in the wilderness, He was preparing himself for the tough mission that God had sent him to accomplish. Therefore, He wanted to focus on God and rely on Him for strength and wisdom before He carried out the task ahead, dying for our sins.

There are many more reasons to fast. However as a general practice, fasting can be done simply because we want to worship and spend time with God just as Prophetess Anna who chose to spend over half of her life praying and fasting:

> *And there was a prophetess, Anna the daughter of Phanuel,*
> *of the tribe of Asher. She was advanced in years and had*
> *lived with her husband seven years after her marriage,*
> *and then as a widow to the age of eighty-four. She never left*
> *the temple, serving night and day with fastings and prayers.*
> *(Luke 2:36-37).*

However, we should be very careful and aware that fasting is not a practice to get God to do something for us, but for us to be transformed and strengthened while focusing our total dependence on Him. When this happens, our situation can be transformed. However, if we fast for something outside God's will, it does not make God reconsider anything. What fasting does is that it changes us. That is why we give up things that matter to our flesh and focus on Him who matters most.

In addition to the spiritual benefits that fasting primarily bestows upon us, this sacrifice has some health benefits. It is important to know that fasting is not a weight loss tool. It is a spiritual tool that connects us with God. Yes, it is possible to lose weight while fasting; however, it is not the goal for Christian believers. After fasting, we should be detoxed of any impurities in both the spiritual and physical body because we do not always eat as healthy as we should, and we do not always act and think as spiritually as we should. Therefore, we should at times give up certain foods to reboot our spirituality, which also boosts our immune system, and metabolism. As we do this, our bodies will look healthier and glow as Daniel and his friends did:

> "Daniel said to him, "Please test us for ten days. Give us nothing but vegetables to eat. And give us only water to drink. Then compare us with the young men who eat the king's food. See how we look. After that, do what you want to." So the guard agreed. He tested them for ten days. After the ten days they looked healthy and well fed. In fact, they looked better than any of the young men who ate the king's food (Daniel 1: 12-15).

Many Churches, Christian, and even nonbelievers are now participating in what is known as the Daniel fast. They are noticing the same positive results that Daniel and his friends acquired, of feeling and looking better. The same results including having less sickness symptoms are being achieved today by eating vegetables. Many detox plans today resulting in clear and smooth skins are also basing their diets on eating just fruits and vegetables because of their nutritious values. Eating raw vegetables and fruits is more nutritious. Following is one way of eating greens differently:

- 1 bunch kale
- I/2 cup roasted nuts of your choice
- 1/2 cup dried cherries or cranberries
- 2 ounces soft goat cheese
- 4 tablespoons olive oil
- 1/2 large onion caramelized onions
- 1 1/2 tablespoons white wine vinegar
- 1 tablespoon smooth Dijon mustard
- 1 1/2 teaspoons honey
- salt and freshly ground black pepper to taste

Slice red or white onion and cook on medium heat until golden and let cool.

Rinse and thoroughly dry kale and chop.

Pour 1 tablespoons olive oil to kale and massage into the kale until it's coated.

WE ARE WHAT WE EAT AND DO:

Add crumbled goat cheese, nuts and onions and dried fruit to kale

For the dressing: Mix Dijon mustard, raw honey and ACV with the mother

Slowly add 2 tablespoons olive oil as you whisk

Pour dressing, salt and pepper to kale salad and mix.

May add chopped lean protein for a heartier meal.

Let sit for at least 20 minutes. ENJOY!

It was long discovered that calorie restrictions can increase the lifespan of certain animals. In recent discoveries there are suggestions that intermittent fasting can provide the same health benefits to human beings, including the following scientifically proven benefits:

- produce weight loss
- lower triglyceride levels
- improve our metabolic disease risk markers
- reduce insulin resistance
- turn us into efficient fat burners
- Gets rids of toxins
- boost our level of human growth hormone, also known as the fitness hormone
- normalize hunger hormones
- reduce inflammation and lessen free radical damage
- improve brain function

In recent health observations, fasting has also been shown to boost production of proteins that help protect our neuro-muscular system from breaking down, which would otherwise result in changes associated with Alzheimer's and Parkinson's disease.

One does not have to be a fasting Christian to know that fasting has physiological in addition to spiritual benefits. It has been practiced throughout the world since the beginning of time. Nothing God commands us to do is for naught.

The bible does not specify how long we should fast but offers several illustrations of godly people who fasted. As followers of Christ, Jesus apparently expects us to fast. When He gave us instructions on how to fast, He did not say IF we fast, but said WHEN we fast, assuming that we would already be fasting:

> *And when you fast, don't make it obvious, as the hypocrites do, for they try to look miserable and disheveled so people will admire them for their fasting. I tell you the truth that is the only reward they will ever get (Mathew 6:16-18).*

What I now know

In this chapter what I found most interesting is:

_____

_____

_____

_____

_____

~~~~

From this chapter I intend to do the following toward healthier eating:

_____

_____

_____

_____

_____

CHAPTER THIRTEEN

DIETING

Accept him whose faith is weak, without passing judgment on disputable matters. One man's faith allows him to eat everything, but another man, whose faith is weak, eats only vegetables. The man who eats everything must not look down on him who does not, and the man who does not eat everything must not condemn the man who does, for God has accepted him. Who are you to judge someone else's servant? To his own master he stands or falls. And he will stand, for the Lord is able to make him stand. One man considers one day more sacred than another; another man considers every day alike. Each one should be fully convinced in his own mind. He who regards one day as special, does so to the Lord. He who eats meat, eats to the Lord, for he gives thanks to God; and he who abstains, does so to the Lord and gives thanks to God (Romans 14:1-6)

We choose what we want to eat or not to eat and select certain foods over others for personal reasons. Most reasons are based on our beliefs, be they religious or health related. Whatever the reason, the Word tells us not to judge but to respect the individuals and their food decisions. Although the cited verse above referred to the judgment that was going on between the Gentiles and the Jews with regards to eating the right foods, the same issues can be said about us today. Sometimes we might judge those we think are not making an effort to eat healthy, assuming that is the reason they are overweight or sick. We are called not to judge. Eating healthy all the time is very difficult and requires a lot of discipline, finances, time and motivation. As we now know, being healthy also encompasses built-in factors that require added effort to overcome. Hence, we cannot and should not be opinionated about anyone based on how one looks or what one is eating. Dieting is an individualized effort whose focus should be self-directed:

> Each one should test his own actions. Then he can take pride
> in himself, without comparing himself to somebody else
> (Galatians 6:4).

We, therefore, cannot talk about food and health and neglect to address the issue of dieting. Yet if anyone is eagerly anticipating reading about diets in this section, there might be some great disappointments. Well, first let's figure out what might be going on in our minds when we hear the word "diet." Some of us cringe at this word as it brings back memories of unpleasant dieting experiences. With some of us it might bring a smile as we remember how much better we looked and felt after the dieting experience got us to our weight goal. Either way, the word "diet" is usually associated with generally undesirable connotation phrases like: losing weight, starving, watching what we eat, cutting down on the foods we like, drinking more water, eating healthy, eating fewer sweets, or watching our waistline. According to the Oxford Dictionary, a diet is: *A special course of food to which a person restricts themselves, either to lose weight or for medical reasons.*

Whatever the reason anyone decides to diet, it is a difficult endeavor. That is why even people who should diet because of medical reasons have a difficult go at it. Dieting does not only apply to people who "look" like they should diet because they are overweight. For example, there are people walking around with fat in their veins that could cause serious health hazards such as heart attack or stroke, who also need to be on low-calorie- and fat-free diets. There are also some people who have diseases related to kidneys who are required to give up salt or high protein meals. We do not see and know what is going on in anyone's body and lives and how we would handle the situation if we were in the same shoe:

> *Let no one therefore judge you in eating, or in drinking, or with respect to a feast day or a new moon or a Sabbath day (Colossians 2:16).*

WE ARE WHAT WE EAT AND DO:

As previously mentioned, more factors such as genetics and hormones can contribute to how our bodies react and process food. That is why some of us tend to gain weight or some of us lose more weight faster than others. On the flip side with those mentioned earlier with high metabolism, there are some people who have predisposed genetic components that lead to high resting metabolic rates. High resting metabolic rates can cause people to gain weight easily. Nevertheless, as also previously stressed, the One who is in us gives us power to overcome anything that the devil brings to us to destroy us:

> *Behold, I give you the authority to trample on serpents and scorpions, and over all the power of the enemy, and nothing shall by any means hurt you (Luke 10:19).*

To do this we need wisdom and knowledge. There is no one best diet that can be given as a stamp of approval because there are so many factors that affect and make diet plans different for each individual. Eating healthy and exercising are the best methods for us to get all nutrients needed by the body and lose weight in a safe manner. That is why some of us might have been disappointed when the diet that worked for our friend, sister or that famous celebrity did not work for us. We should at all times consult with our healthcare providers before we start on any diet program. This will help in identifying any medical conditions which might need to be closely monitored while on diet. In some cases, if losing weight is hormonally related, such as when having thyroid disease, one might find it a bit difficult to lose weight, and this can also be discovered during medical consultation. When this is true, taking care of the medical issue becomes a high priority and in turn may help with the weight problem once fixed. Though diet plans are not being provided, for the purpose of this book it would be negligent not to be informative of the unhealthy ways of dieting.

As noted in the definition of diet, when one is dieting for weight loss, consideration must be given as to the length of time one is on the diet. For example, if one is on a calorie reduction diet, the duration on the diet should be limited to support the goals defined for the weight loss. Dieting is not supposed to be long term, and if continuously sustained, increased weight loss can occur causing malnourishment. Diets that are long term are usually medical or life time changes such as being a vegetarian and those include giving up certain indicated foods. Not everything that is called a diet is safe and healthy. We should make sure we consult experts on the right diet program and it should be individualized. While searching for the best way to go for us, here is what we should be cognizant of in types of diets that might be unreliable. Those that:

- Promote quick weight loss
- Limit food selections

- Use testimonials from famous people or tie the diet to a well-known city
- Bill themselves as cure-alls
- Often recommend expensive supplements
- Do not attempt to change eating habits permanently
- Are generally critical of and skeptical about scientific community
- Claim there is no need to exercise
- Food replacements with supplements

Losing weight in a healthy manner should be about change of life style. When attempting a diet regiment, focus should be on long term results which can be achieved primarily by a life-time life-style change to healthier living. Short term goals of dieting help us get motivated because, as impatient humans beings, we sometimes tend to give up when we do not see immediate results. However, a short term healthy diet, if correctly applied, should motivate us when we see those pounds, glucose, and cholesterol go down. We then can slowly adjust our healthy eating to fit our long term life style.

Although when we diet we are supposed to mainly focus on our health, it would be deceiving to say that for most of us our looks are not considered the utmost priority. Body image and eating disorders haunt many of us more than the concern of eating the right thing. It is even harder when looks are made to be everything in today's Diasporian society. How we look instead of what we eat has caused some of us to do whatever it takes to have "that look." These issues do not get enough attention except through weight loss plans. Although many of the weight loss methods are actually good and helpful, for Christians they do not address what the Bible has to say about health and our bodies, as well as nutrition and eating habits.

As we worry about being overweight and the associated health risks, being in Diaspora we raise children in a culture that values looking slim like a runway model as being beautiful. Because of this our kids may adopt under-eating habits that can lead to harmful health issues. There are risks associated with over-dieting to the point where one is malnourished. Societal issues such as peer pressure, health messages from media, and desire for independence may put our kids at risk for such diseases as Anorexia Nervosa or Bulimia. Anorexia Nervosa begins with a desire to lose weight which becomes an obsession. People with AV are genuinely petrified of being overweight, and see themselves as obese even when they are thin to the bone. They begin a cycle of willful starvation and compulsive exercising to burn off calories. Bulimics are also preoccupied with feeling fat and begin to under-eat. With prolonged dieting, they can experience an intense hunger and craving for food, especially junk food. Once they begin to eat they find it hard to stop, which causing them to feel guilty and very uncomfortable, and then they induce vomiting, which becomes a cycle of binging and purging.

WE ARE WHAT WE EAT AND DO:

As we encourage our kids to eat age appropriate healthy diets and keep active, we should be careful NOT TO OVER-EMPHASIZE fat-reduced diets during childhood as they may create negative body image issues, low self-esteem and eating disorders. Again, when we eat together as a family, we are able to monitor what we put on our kids' plates and how they eat.

Following are some famous quotes to consider that might bring us some enlightenment concerning eating healthy and maybe a few chuckles.

You don't have to cook fancy or complicated masterpieces — just good food from fresh ingredients~. Julia Child

Don't eat anything your great-great grandmother wouldn't recognize as food. There are a great many food-like items in the supermarket your ancestors wouldn't recognize as food…"~ Michael Polland

He that takes medicine and neglects diet wastes, the skills of the physician. ~Chinese proverb

The doctor of the future will no longer treat the human frame with drugs, but rather will cure and prevent disease with nutrition. ~Thomas Edison

If hunger is not the problem, then eating is not the solution ~. Anonymous

Finally, in Zimbabwe we have a saying: *Ukama igasva,*
hunozadziswa nekuday - a relationship is
not complete when food has not been shared.

What I now know

In this chapter what I found most interesting is:

_____

_____

_____

_____

_____

~~~~

From this chapter I intend to do the following toward healthier eating:

_____

_____

_____

_____

_____

CHAPTER FOURTEEN

NATURAL FUNCTIONING FOODS

For the Lord your God is bringing you into a good land, a
land of brooks of water, of fountains and springs, flowing out
in the valleys and hills, A land of wheat and barley, of vines
and fig trees and pomegranates, a land of olive trees and
honey (Deuteronomy 8:8).

Is it not just an awesome and wonderful thing knowing that our God is not a God of randomness but that He is purposeful and that everything He does for us is for our own good? He would not send us to a place to harm us and leave us there alone without instructions for healthy living. Among other foods, certain foods are depicted as being in a land of prosperity: wheat, barley, vines of grapes, figs, pomegranates, olives and honey. All these are known to have great health benefits. What is in these foods, and what makes them so special?

They are some of what we know today as functional foods. Functional foods are foods with a potential to function in a health-promotion and maintenance or disease prevention capacity. These foods offer great potential to improve health and/or help prevent certain illnesses when taken as part of a balanced diet in a healthy lifestyle. The subject of health claims on certain foods is becoming increasingly important to the point that there is a broad consensus about the need to regulate systems that protect consumers. Though established from the beginning of time, more foods are being recognized as "super foods" with healing power today.

Honey is one of the most nutritious and healthiest natural foods. It is known for its natural sweetness and great taste, but it is also full of riboflavin, thiamine, pantothenic acid, pyridoxine, niacin, calcium, copper, iron, magnesium, manganese, phosphorus, potassium, zinc, and vitamin C. Beyond that, natural raw honey has a lot more health benefits, both nutritionally and medicinally. In the ancient times, it was used in embalming fluid and to dress wounds. Today, there are many home remedies that advocate the use of raw natural honey for many ailments.

It would be to our benefit to keep a jar or two of natural raw honey in the house; one for health inside our bodies, and the other to apply outside (See APPENDIX B for more honey benefits):

> *Eat honey, my son, for it is good; honey from the comb is sweet to your taste (Proverb 24:13).*

It is important to note here that as healthy as honey is, **it is not safe for pregnant women, during breast feeding and for infants under 1 year old.** According to the US Food and Drug

Administration honey can contain the Clostridium botulinum organism that could cause serious illness or death. The botulism bacteria spores are found in dust and soil and make their way into honey. Because older people have developed natural defenses in intestines that prevent the growth of botulism spores, they are able to defend themselves from the toxins and infection. However, cooked honey in foods such as cereals is safe for infants. In diabetics, honey should be used sparingly as it is still a sugar that can raise glucose levels in the blood.

Whole natural wheat and barley are healthy grains that have large amounts of fiber, minerals and vitamins. In their natural unprocessed state, these grains contain 30% of our recommended daily fiber intake. Wheat has high levels of manganese and magnesium, vitamin B1, B2, B3, E, folic acid, calcium, phosphorus, zinc, copper, and iron. Barley contains copper, manganese, selenium, vitamin B1 and B3, chromium, phosphorus, magnesium. Some health benefits from these minerals and vitamins help in reducing the symptoms of arthritis. High fiber diet helps with digestion to eliminate toxins in our bodies and in turn reduce risks of colon cancer. The bulkiness of fiber also helps lower cholesterol and loss of weight. Fiber has low glycemic index which helps regulate type-2 diabetes if eaten regularly. A diet rich in wheat and barley can also increase energy level.

Besides the well-known product of wine from grapes, this fruit contains nutritious compounds called flavonoids, which are believed to reduce the risk of blood clots and protect our bodies from damage by the toxins found in the bad cholesterol (LDL). As antioxidants, grapes may provide protection against cardiovascular disease, particularly in women.

Figs are sweet fruits, eaten either dried or fresh. They are high in potassium, a mineral that is used in treatment of high blood pressure and stroke prevention as well as nerve, muscle and chemical functions. High also in dietary fiber, figs help with digestion. They also contain calcium, which may help preserve bone density, heart, nerve and blood clotting functions. The leaves of a fig tree are not typically eaten but can be made into an extract, which may help lower insulin levels in diabetics.

Today, pomegranates are trendy and considered super-foods, particularly in a juice format. This fruit is rich in antioxidants, which prevent bad cholesterol (LDL) from damaging our blood vessels and help prevent blood clots by keeping blood platelets from clumping together. Pomegranates may also help reduce the risk of breast cancer and lessen the symptoms of arthritis.

Olives, in their best format as extra-virgin oil, contain many of the antioxidants that are thought to protect against the oxidation (making them more dangerous) of bad cholesterol. They are also high in monounsaturated fatty acids, which are called "the healing fats" because they lower the effects of "bad"
cholesterol while raising "good" cholesterol (HDL) levels. Olive oil

is high in vitamin E and is thought to protect against colon cancer and is helpful to fight stomach ailments.

In addition to these Biblically mentioned foods, there are so many other foods that are considered healthy and worth incorporating in our daily diets or keeping at hand. A very good example of a versatile beneficial food is apple cider vinegar (ACV). ACV is best taken and most beneficial when it is "with the mother." Any other way would be a waste of money and time. ACV with the mother has wonderful and great benefits for inside and outside our bodies. Why with the mother? Because in this form, it is raw, organic, unpasteurized, and the strand-like sediments that float or settle at the bottom when not shaken is Mother Nature's perfect food. As a healthcare practitioner, I have observed some of my patients lose weight and control their diabetes. For weight loss ACV has been shown to help suppress appetite or make one feel full. For diabetes it has been shown to lower blood sugar. Success has also been noted in the reduction of cholesterol level, relief from stiff arthritic joints, relief from itchy scalp, and help with indigestion. That being said, its acidity can make it difficult for most of us to take. However, it can be enjoyed as a cold drink by mixing:

- 1 - 2 tsps ACV in 8 oz water to taste.
- 1-2 tsps Organic Honey, 100% Maple Syrup, Blackstrap Molasses OR 4 drops herb Stevia (for diabetics) to taste
- 1 - 2tsps fresh squeezed lemon

WE ARE WHAT WE EAT AND DO:

It can also be enjoyed as hot beverage at breakfast:
- Cup of hot water
- 2 to 3 cinnamon sticks
- 4 cloves

Steep 20 minutes or more.

Before serving add ACV and raw honey or stevia to taste

ACV with the mother can also be used to make a delicious salad dressing as follows:

- 1/3 cup raw apple cider vinegar with the mother
- 1/4 cup extra-virgin olive oil
- ¼ cup flax seed oil
- 1 minced garlic clove
- 1 tablespoon Dijon mustard
- 1/2 freshly squeezed lemon juice
- 2 tablespoons raw honey, or as needed for sweetness
- cayenne pepper (optional) to taste

Combine all of the ingredients in a glass jar, then seal the lid and shake until the honey dissolves and the ingredients are well combined. Adjust the flavor to taste, if necessary.

For best flavor, allow the dressing to marinate for at least 30 minutes before serving over salad.

Store leftovers in the fridge for up to a week, and shake well before serving each time. ENJOY!

Besides adding flavor and an aromatic richness to our food, the use of spices and herbs has traditional historic habits in many African and Eastern countries, which are now increasingly being adopted in the Western world. Must-haves to keep in the kitchen and to use all the time are:

ginger	cayenne	pepper	cinnamon
turmeric	garlic	ginseng	sage
rosemary	green tea		

Drinking a freshly squeezed lemon in green tea with added cinnamon, raw honey, ACV with the mother and an optional dash of cayenne pepper can start us off with healthy zing in the morning. Following is a healthy kale bean soup recipe with a list of beneficial ingredients:

- 1 tablespoon olive oil
- 8 large garlic cloves, crushed or minced
- 1 medium yellow onion, chopped
- 1 medium carrot, diced into 1/4-inch cubes
- 1 cup diced celery
- 4 small tomatoes chopped
- 4 cups chopped raw kale, rinsed stems removed
- 4 cups low-fat, low-sodium chicken or vegetable broth
- 2 (15 ounce) cans white beans or beans without draining
- 2 tsp dried thyme
- 2 tsp dried sage

- Salt & pepper to taste

Pre-cooked lean meat (turkey, chicken or beef) optional

In a large pot heat the olive oil, add garlic, onion and tomatoes, celery and carrots,

Sauté till soft.

Add kale and sauté, stirring, until wilted.

Add 3 cups of broth

Add 1 can of beans reserving 1 cup and all of the herbs, salt and pepper.

Simmer 5 minutes.

In a blender or food processor or by hand, mix the remaining beans with the broth until smooth.

Stir into soup to thicken. Simmer 15 minutes and ladle into Bowls. ENJOY!

Recipe Benefits (See APPENDIX C for more functional foods)

- **Olive oil**- lowers risk of heart disease, lowers cholesterol, protects against blood clotting, controls blood sugar
- **Garlic-**lowers risk of heart disease, high blood pressure, and cancer, lowers cholesterol,
- **Onions-**Vitamins B6 and C, Cancer, protects against blood clotting, antibiotic effects
- **Carrots-** Vitamin A, skin, vision, antioxidant
- **Celery-**Vitamin A, C, hydration, antioxidant, natural salt
- **Tomatoes-** lower risk of heart disease and cancer, prevent DNA damage, protect against blood clotting, lower inflammation, reduce fluid retention

- **Kale-** Vitamins A, C and K, fiber, antioxidant
- **White Beans-**antioxidants, good source of fiber and protein, low glycemic index, regulate fat storage
- **Thyme-** germ killer, stomach problems
- **Sage-**digestive problems, depression, painful menstruation

What I now know

In this chapter what I found most interesting is:

_____

_____

_____

_____

_____

~~~~

From this chapter I intend to do the following toward healthier eating:

_____

_____

_____

_____

_____

CHAPTER FIFTEEN

DIETARY SUPPLEMENTS

And on the banks, on both sides of the river, there will grow all kinds of trees for food. Their leaves will not wither, nor their fruit fail, but they will bear fresh fruit every month because the, water for them flows from the sanctuary. Their fruit will be for food, and their leaves for healing." (Ezekiel 47:12).

When God created us He also provided us with everything we could ever think or dream of including all the nutrition our wonderfully made bodies need inside out. He gave us plants that provide us with an abundance of both nutrition and healing features, which our bodies need to fully function and stay healthy. Being the imperfect humans we are, not all of us always eat the way we should to keep our bodies at their optimum. So how do we overcome the problem of not getting all the nutrients we need in the foods we eat? Most nutritionists and dieticians recommend taking dietary supplements. But what are dietary supplements, and do we really need them every day?

WE ARE WHAT WE EAT AND DO:

The human body requires various vitamins and minerals on a daily basis to keep alive, healthy and functioning. Dietary supplements provide proper cell production, chemical balance, and functioning of our bodies. Their main purpose is to boost overall health and energy, provide immune system support, reduce the risks of illness and age-related conditions, support the healing process during disease, and help correct deficiency based illnesses. Dietary supplements are there to enhance any incomplete diet. They are intended to supplement the diet and provide nutrients but not to replace the food. As such, there are so many supplements and their uses are also so vast that it is impossible to go through all of them. In this book only the basics of supplements will be addressed (see APPENDIX C for some more dietary supplement functions).

Dietary supplements are found naturally in plants and animals. They can also be made in the labs, which makes them synthetic or artificial. Minerals come from the soil absorbed through water by plants or eaten by animals. Vitamins are divided into two groups, the water-soluble which are B-complex and vitamin C; and the fat-soluble are A, D, E, and K. Water-soluble vitamins dissolve in water and pass through the body quickly, meaning that the body needs them on a regular basis. Fat-soluble vitamins should be taken with food that contains fat to be best used up. They are stored in the body's fatty tissue, meaning that they can remain in the body for a long period of time.

Vitamins and minerals are most easily digested with food. Our body uses vitamins in specific amounts based on our gender, age, and health conditions. One of the most significant health issues is that related to digestive conditions due to absorption capabilities. Vitamins cannot be absorbed without minerals, and some minerals are best absorbed with certain vitamins. For example, iron is best absorbed if taken with vitamin C. Vitamins tend to work synergistically, meaning that they work together in order to be effective. For instance, vitamin E requires some of the vitamin B-complex and selenium and zinc minerals to be best absorbed. Some minerals may not be absorbed or may inhibit each other. For instant, iron is best absorbed in the presence of Vitamin C, and Vitamin C should not be taken with aspirin, as it can irritate the stomach and limit absorption. Large amounts of zinc may deplete the body of the copper mineral, while too much calcium adversely affects the magnesium levels in the body. So, there is a lot to consider when taking vitamins and minerals.

Herbal supplements are substances only found in plants that have notable health effects in the body. They have been used for centuries and continue to be used in many traditional health systems for nutritious and medicinal purposes. They are actually the basis for some of today's common medicines. For example, willow bark tea has been used for centuries to control fever, and pharmaceutical companies eventually identified the chemical in willow bark that reduces fever and used that information to produce aspirin. A quarter of all drugs today have been derived directly from plant sources, including Codeine (from poppy seeds) and Paclitaxel (Taxol), a drug for ovarian and breast cancer (from the Pacific Yew tree).

Historically, people have used herbal medicines to prevent illness, cure infection, reduce fever, and heal wounds. Some herbal medicines can also treat constipation, ease pain, or act as relaxants or stimulants. Research on some herbs and plant products has shown that they may have some of the same effects that conventional medicines do. Examples are Omega-3 fatty acids that may help to lower triglyceride levels, 5-HTP, a nutritious supplement for the brain, or St. John's Wort as antidepressants.

If we don't practice sound nutritious eating habits, over time we can develop nutrient deficiencies. Nutrient deficiencies can lead to serious medical problems, such as anemia, bone fragility, poor immune system function, and nervous system abnormalities. These health issues can, of course, be reversed or corrected if identified on time. Specific types of dietary supplements can also help reduce risks for certain types of diseases and medical conditions. For example, folic acid taken during pregnancy reduces the risk of the unborn baby from developing nervous system birth defects.

As previously mentioned, there are medical conditions and individual circumstances that may make it difficult for our bodies to efficiently obtain the vitamins and minerals from regular diet. For example, behaviors such as overeating can inhibit nutrition digestion and absorption. Sedentary life styles can also decrease absorption of nutrients. Conditions such as being allergic to dairy products such as milk can make it difficult to gain adequate levels of vitamin D and calcium from regular diet. In these situations, dietary supplements can fill unmet nutritious needs, but should not be taken as food. Dietary supplements containing these needed substances can help ensure that the needed nutrient are met, thereby decreasing risks for diseases such as osteoporosis. We can find out what our bodies are lacking by consulting our healthcare providers especially if we are symptomatic.

How safe then are these dietary supplements? As a matter of fact, not all herbs and supplements are safe. Just because most of them are naturally found or that we make them in our bodies does not guarantee their safety if not taken appropriately. In addition, it is by no means safe to forgo our conventional medical treatment and rely only on dietary supplement. Therefore, if unsure about the safety of a supplement or herb, we should talk to a healthcare provider, pharmacist, or dietitian. Most of all, we should inform our primary healthcare provider of any dietary supplements we are using.

When using dietary supplements, we should keep in mind that since they are chemically based, like conventional medicines, they may cause side effects or trigger allergies. For instance vitamin C may cause gas, bloating or diarrhea, iron can cause constipation, and vitamins may cause nausea if taken on an empty stomach in some people. We should also be aware that dietary supplements can interact with prescription and nonprescription medicines or other supplements we might be taking at the same time. Taking more dietary supplements is not necessarily better because toxicity can occur. For instance, while excess water soluble vitamins can be eliminated when we sweat or go to the bathroom, fat soluble vitamins last longer in the system, and therefore, if taken in higher doses, can cause overdose effects. In addition, for those with kidney or liver diseases some herbs may not be efficiently eliminated from the body and therefore cause overdose effects.

Lastly, not all dietary supplements are created equal. How well they work or any side effects they cause may differ based on manufacturer or brand name. How then do we know which supplements work well and which ones to pick off the shelf from all those hundreds of different multivitamins on the market, with some even found in the dollar store? When we look at the labels of the supplements of the same product, for example one labeled multivitamins, we might notice that the content and amount of vitamins listed might be different. The following four suggestions can be considered when deciding which supplements to buy.

First we should consider the **amounts** of vitamins and minerals listed on the bottle based on personal needs. Buying too much will be a waste and any extra will end up going down the toilet or being potentially dangerous. With too little, we would not be getting the benefits we need or our money's worth. Second, we should consider the **type** of vitamins and minerals. For instance vitamin D comes in D2 and D3 format. D3 is better because it is similar to the type we make in our bodies and thereby is also better processed in our bodies. Third, we should consider the **quality and price** of the supplements. For instance, we should focus on whether a multivitamin actually contains the claimed amounts of what it should and none of what it shouldn't. Of course unless you are in the lab watching the vitamin making process, it would be difficult for us to tell by just reading the label. Unfortunately, the general rule of thumb is to go natural and expensive, meaning the cheaper it is, the less likely it is good quality. Fourth, we should buy according **to specific health needs**. There should not be any need to take a multivitamin and multi minerals when all you need is vitamin B12 or iron. We should also not forget to consider our age, gender, diet, life style and symptoms. Generally men and menopausal women would not need to take multivitamin that contain iron, unless they have iron deficiency or have a health condition such as anemia.

We all know at least one person who takes vitamins, minerals or herbs every day. We also know some people who don't believe in dietary supplements. The question then remains: do we really need to be taking all those pills every day? Well, yes and no. We discussed the purpose of dietary supplements that they complement, enhance, or add to what is lacking. If nothing is lacking nothing needs to be supplemented. Thus the saying, "If it's not broke, don't fix it." On the other hand, if our diet is not as wholesome as it should be, yes, we probably need to supplement, but only after we know what it is we need to supplement. Of course, what we should really be doing is improving the overall diet because supplements alone won't magically fix the problem. If our diet actually is really good, no, we most likely don't need to take any supplements.

What we should mostly understand about supplements is that we cannot replace daily recommended servings of fruits and vegetables with daily vitamins. A healthful diet is the most preferred way to obtain the nutrients our body needs. At least five servings per day of fruits and vegetables are recommended, as well as the inclusion of whole grains in the diet. When we look at our plates, the more colorful it is with lots of combination of foods types, the more likely it contains more vitamins and minerals. Nutrients from food sources are more efficiently utilized by the body than isolated supplemental substances. For instance, fresh fruit and leafy green vegetable juice could be used to provide concentrated amounts of particular nutrients, such as vitamins A, B, C, and K to the diet

Another example of a well enjoyed common dish back home loaded with multivitamins and minerals made from pumpkin, peanut butter and milk is *nhopi* (pumpkin porridge):

- 1 cup cornmeal (vitamin B-complex, zinc, calcium and iron)
- ½ teaspoon brown sugar:
- 1 cup water

- 1 cup low fat milk (if grass fed cow milk vitamins A, B2, B12, D, iodine, phosphorus, calcium, pantothenic acid, selenium, biotin)
- 3 tablespoons peanut butter: (biotin, copper, manganese, vitamins B, B3, molybdenum, folate, vitamin E, phosphorus)
- 1/2 pumpkin, (or butternut squash) peeled, cooked and mashed and salted (beta and alpha- carotene, potassium, pantothenic acid, magnesium, and vitamins C and E)

Put water to a large pan with pumpkins and bring to a boil
Then add the cornmeal (maize meal) and stir frequently
until you form a thick paste
Add milk, sugar and peanut butter
Stir everything together to ensure all the ingredients are
 incorporated
Continue cooking for a few minutes and add a little water
if the mixture is too thick… ENJOY!

That being said, we are in Diaspora where we have identified barriers to obtaining affordable healthy foods. It is said Americans have the poorest eating habits in the world. This is not because of the famous burgers and fries, pizza or any other junk food. It is because of the food production practices. Modern farming practices that include the way the soil is stripped of nutrients give us foods that are not as healthy as they used to be.

WE ARE WHAT WE EAT AND DO:

It has been shown that the amount of minerals, particularly trace minerals, may be decreasing in foods due to mineral depletion of the soil caused by unsustainable farming practices and soil erosion. Gone are the days of crop rotation that helped manage soil fertility and also reduce soil diseases and soil-dwelling insects. Instead pesticides and other modern approaches are used to produce food for mass consumption. As previously discussed, how and where we get our food matters, and how we prepare and store our food matters.

What I now know

In this chapter what I found most interesting is:

_____

_____

_____

_____

_____

~~~~

From this chapter I intend to do the following toward healthier eating:

_____

_____

_____

_____

_____

CHAPTER SIXTEEN

WHAT'S ON OUR PLATE?

*So, whether you eat or drink, or whatever you do, do all to
the glory of God (1 Corinthians 10:31).*

Whatever is on our plates, we ought to feel very blessed
and give thanks to our Lord with appreciation that there are
others who go without any food. As Christians, we will be
walking in the footsteps of Jesus as He showed to bless our food:

*And as they were eating, Jesus took bread, and blessed it,
and broke it, and gave it to the disciples, and said, Take, eat;
this is my body (Matthew 26:26).*

Being fortunate enough to have food, we should also be aware
of what it is we are dishing on our plates. All food groups come
down to five basic components: water, vitamins and minerals,
carbohydrates, proteins, and fats. Since vitamins and minerals
were previously discussed as dietary supplements, only the other
four groups will be addressed in this chapter.

Eat whatever is sold in the meat market without raising any question on the ground of conscience. For "the earth is the Lord's, and everything in it." (1Corinthians 10:25-26).

Water

Then measure out a jar of water for each day, and drink it at set times (Ezekiel 4:11).

Water is a very important nutrient for our physical and spiritual livelihood. In the Bible, water is mostly referred to as the Living Water that gives us eternal life. This is symbolic to our earthly life as the water is also very valuable to our existence. As Jesus said:

But whoever drinks the water I give him will never thirst. Indeed, the water I give him will become in him a spring of water welling up to eternal life (John 4:14).

Yes, indeed, water gives us life here and beyond. It is the basis of all our bodily function, and we therefore need it to survive here on earth. Our body is made up to 60% of water of which the brain and heart are 73% water, the lungs 83% water, the skin 64% water, muscles and kidneys 79%, and even bones 31% water. We can now see how without water, our body would shrivel and die.

125

WE ARE WHAT WE EAT AND DO:

When we drink water, it is reabsorbed in the large intestine before it is eliminated mostly as urine or sweat. The water which is reabsorbed serves a number of essential functions to sustain our bodies and as a vital nutrient to the life of every cell. The carbohydrates and proteins that our bodies use as food are metabolized and transported by water into the bloodstream, while it helps burn fat and build muscle. Water regulates our internal body temperature when we sweat. It assists in flushing out waste mainly through urination. It also acts as a shock absorber for the brain, spinal cord, and fetus, forms saliva, keeps our skin healthy and elastic, hair hydrated, and lubricates and cushions joints. Water maintains the volume and viscosity of blood, which prevents blood from thickening, reducing the risk of hypertension and cardiovascular diseases.

For practical day to day use, drinking water on an empty stomach facilitates its easy absorption by the body. Drinking it 30 minutes before each meal makes us feel fuller, without having consumed any calories, thereby compelling us to eat less. Drinking two glasses of water just after waking up helps stimulate the peristaltic muscles and boosts blood circulation.

Although we can get water in some foods we eat and drink such as tomatoes, celery, watermelons, and tea, we still need to consume it in its natural state. To prevent dehydration, we should replace the water our body loses through normal everyday functions when going to the bathroom, sweating or breathing. It is recommended that we drink 2 liters of water a day, that's eight

8oz glasses. There are times when we need to drink more water than usual. Our bodies need this extra water when the weather is hot, during and after physical activities, when we are sick to help flush out toxins and reduce fever, and when we have diarrhea or vomiting, to avoid dehydration.

Carbohydrates

Take wheat and barley, beans and lentils, millet and spelt; put them in a storage jar and use them to make bread for yourself... (Ezekiel 4:9a).

These mentioned foods are carbohydrates or "carbs" as we commonly call them. Carbohydrates are traditionally the largest serving on our plates, though we now know better. There are three main types of carbohydrate in the food we eat: starches - known as complex carbohydrates, sugars, and fiber. Foods high in starch originate from produce like peas, beans, lentil, corn, potatoes, and grains such as oats, barley and rice. Final products from carbohydrates include but are not limited to our beloved pasta, bread and *sadza*.

Starches are made up of three parts:

Bran–is the outer hard shell of grain, providing the most fiber and most of the B vitamins and minerals.

Germ-is the next layer packed with nutrients including essential fatty acids and vitamin E

Endosperm-is the soft part in the center of the grain containing starch.

Grains can be divided into whole grain or refined grain. When we eat the whole grain food, we have eaten bran, germ, and endosperm, therefore, we would be getting all of the nutrients that the whole grain has to offer. Refined grain foods contain only the endosperm or the starchy part so if we eat this part only, we would be missing out on a lot of vitamins and minerals.

The next type of carbs is sugar and there are two main types of sugar in our diets. There is the naturally occurring sugar such as that found in milk or fruit. Then there is the added sugar such as that added during food processing. An example is that of fruit canned in heavy corn syrup or sugar added when making cookies. Added sugars are processed sugars and therefore contain no nutritious benefit.

Fiber only comes from plants, so there is no fiber in any animal products such as milk, eggs, meat, poultry, and fish. There are two types of fiber, digestible because it is soluble, and indigestible because it is insoluble. Both types can be found in foods such as beans and vegetables. Digestible fiber can be found in citrus fruits, apples, peas, barley, psyllium and oat bran, and non-digestible fiber in wheat bran, whole-wheat flour, nuts and whole-grain foods. It is best to get our fiber from food rather than taking a fiber supplement. Fiber is best taken gradually to prevent stomach irritation, as well as with water to prevent constipation.

The carbohydrates' main purpose is to provide energy for our bodies, used on a cellular level as well as for our body parts. So what happens to carbohydrates when we eat them? Digestion of carbs begins in the mouth when they are moistened and broken down by chewing before going to the stomach. No digestion of carbs happens in the stomach, but hydrochloric acid is produced to kill bacteria. Carbs are then passed on to the small intestine where they are broken down to small sugars. The carbohydrates not digested such as fiber are passed on to the large intestines and removed from the body as stool. In the small intestines, the small sugars are digested to glucose and released to the bloodstream from which they will be carried to our body parts and used as energy. Insulin released from the pancreas helps with the absorption of glucose into our body cells. If there is any excess sugar it is carried to the liver and stored as glycogen. However, the liver's capacity for glycogen is limited, and any excess sugar can cause the liver to expand. **When the liver is full to capacity, the sugar is then returned to the blood in the form of fatty acids. These fatty acids are then transported to every part of our body and are stored as fat.**

Glycemic Index

Not all carbohydrates are created equal and neither are their functions the same. Carbohydrate statuses are associated with a Glycemic Index (GI) rate. This is a measure that offers information about how foods affect blood sugar and insulin in our bodies and are associated with diabetes. Foods that break down quickly, resulting in fast blood glucose surge in the blood stream, have a high GI rating. The higher the GI, the higher the glucose level in the blood and insulin that is released in response. The lower a food's GI, the less it affects blood sugar and, in turn, insulin levels. Some factors that affect GI rating are the food nutrition content, presentation, and condition. For instance, puffed cereals have a much higher GI than the grain they come from. A less ripened fruit such as banana has a lower GI than an overripe one. Higher protein and fat content foods have lower GI than those containing less. Whole orange fruit has a lower GI than in its orange juice condition. How food is processed, cooked and the type of combination in which it is consumed can change the way our body processes the carbohydrates, thereby changing the GI. For instance, with regards to food particle size, the bigger and unprocessed whole grains have a lower GI than when they are made into small fine flower particles. Finally, combining carbohydrates with other foods such as fats and proteins can lower the overall GI of the food.

It is amazing how our Zimbabwean traditional practices of combining carbohydrates with protein support the nutritious GI concepts. For instance *mupunga* or *chibage chine dovi* (peanut butter- Low GI and rice/corn – high GI = overall low GI):

- Brown rice
- Peanut butter 1 tablespoon for each cup of rice

- Water (1/4 cup for each cup of rice).

  Stir water into peanut butter until it becomes a smooth paste and bring to a light simmer.

  Add the rice to the simmering peanut butter.

  Serve while still hot and enjoy as a snack or a meal, Enjoy!

The best way to utilize our carbs is to eat sensibly. The most nutritious way to consume carbohydrates is in their most wholesome state and minimally processed. The general rule of thumb is to stay away from white carbs as they are more likely to be processed or of less nutritious value than their darker counter parts. For example, we should choose brown whole multi grain bread over white bread, brown raw sugar over white sugar, wild or black rice over white rice, or sweet potatoes over white potatoes. Getting acclimated to this eating habit is not always easy if we are accustomed to white bread and white rice, but a gradual ease into unprocessed foods is sometimes key because the change is worth the good health.

The general population loves bread. Most of us can still smell the aroma of warm baking Lobels bread *kumagrosa* (grocery stores), which we ate fresh with margarine melting into the soft warm sliced bread. Beyond the nostalgia and the deliciousness of those memories, the content of that slice was empty hip hugging, rear extending calories. However, as our environment would have it, we would sink our teeth in that deliciousness after burning calories playing *chitsvambe/chitsveru* (tag). Bread is a great food, but to get the most nutrition from it, is to eat it as a whole-grain. It comes in a lot of fun varieties such as containing flaxseed or a variety of nuts. For those of us who like jasmine or basmati rice, it also comes as brown rice. We should also consider wild and black rice. Rice can also be replaced with a healthier barley grain cooked the same way. If *sadza* from corn is what is still preferred after trying other grains, stone ground corn meal with most of its nutritious grain components is ideal to use. And for those of us who cannot go a day without *sadza*, we can experiment with different grains. We should not shy away from s*adza* made from oats and wheat. Back home in Zimbabwe, *sadza* came in different grain formats such as millet, which we can locate in Diaspora. Local Indian groceries carry *zviyo, rukweza, mhunga or rapoko* as bulrush millet or finger millet. Millet contains serotonin which is calming to our moods, magnesium which helps reduce the effects of migraines and heart attacks, and niacin (vitamin B3) which helps lower cholesterol. Other great health millet benefits are high fiber, iron, calcium, protein, low glycemic index antioxidant activity, and it is gluten-free.

Gluten-free!? What is that and what is the craze about gluten-free diet? Basically gluten is a combination of two proteins found chiefly in grains such as wheat, barley and rye. That is what gives dough its elasticity and makes it rise. It has no nutritious value. What it does is it can cause very uncomfortable stomach and skin problems in people who are gluten sensitive to it and in those with celiac disease, an immune related illness that can prevent important nutrients from being absorbed. While a gluten-free diet would be recommended for these disorders, for a person not suffering from these conditions adopting gluten-free diet as a healthy measure would mean giving up a lot of common nutritious foods for no particular reason.

Going back to millet, not only is it one of the most nutritious foods and very easy to digest, it is low in fat most of which is unsaturated fat. Best of all, it can be used to make a healthier light-feeling *sadza* than the processed white corn meal *sadza* version. It may take some getting used to, but if all fails, decreasing the quantity of corn meal *sadza* to the recommended handful serving size and adding more leafy greens and lean protein will be a healthier choice. *Maheu* drink is one of the most memorable millet made drink we grew up drinking on any hot afternoon:

- 2 1/2 liters hot water;
- 1 1/2 liters cold water; and ice cold water to make paste)
  Put the finger millet malt in a large pot.

Add a small amount of cold water to make a smooth paste.

Put the pot on stove top on medium-high heat.

Add the boiling water while stirring simultaneously and
  bring to a boil.

As soon as it is boiling, reduce the heat to a gentle simmer

And allow it to simmer until cooked (about 40 minutes).

When it is cooked, remove from the heat and allow it to
  cool.

Once cooled, slowly add the cold water and stir until you get a thin liquid consistency.

Place the pot of *mahewu* and stir at least once a day

The *mahewu* (finger millet drink) will be ready and fermented within 4 days. CHEERS!

Protein

Every moving thing that lives shall be food for you. And as I gave you the green plants, I give you everything (Genesis 9:3).

Protein is a very important building block of our bones, muscles, cartilage, skin, blood and every cell in our body. It is needed to build and repair our body and to make enzymes, hormones, and other needed body chemicals. Next to water, protein is the second most abundant substance in our body. Most of the time when we think of protein, we picture some kind of meat, however, protein comes in many forms including such foods as beans, nuts, eggs, seeds, and soy. These foods have traditionally always been a healthy part of our diet.

What happens when we eat protein? The process of breaking down protein for digestion starts while we are cooking the meat as the tough connective tissue unfolds and softens. In the mouth, protein is further broken down into smaller pieces to increase surface area for easier digestion. After being passed on to the stomach, with the help of hydrochloric acid, protein is digested into peptides and released into the small intestine. In the small intestine, more enzymes are released to further digest peptides into amino acids. Our body cannot make essential amino acids; therefore, they must come from the food we eat. Because amino acids have very small dimensions, they are able to penetrate the intestinal lining and enter the bloodstream. Once in the bloodstream, amino acids are transported to various tissues, depending on where cell structures need to be created or repaired. **Protein is broken down as needed, and if we eat too much protein, the excess is turned into fatty acids and stored in the liver. When the liver is full, it releases the fatty acids back to the blood stream where they are transported to our body parts and stored as fat.** Protein source greatly influences the amount of time required by individual amino acids to be absorbed.

Lean versions of meat, fish, and chicken, grilled, baked or stewed, are an easy way to incorporate protein into our diet. Our traditional tomato based protein stews are loaded with nutrients from additives like tomatoes and onions. A good example of a very healthy and nutritious protein stew is *kapenta fish* (sardines like fish). *Kapenta* have more health benefits when they are dried and cooked as follows:

- 1 onion, chopped
- 2 or 3 tablespoons oil
- 2 tomatoes, peeled and cut up
- 1 pound dried *kapenta,* washed well, or canned sardines

WE ARE WHAT WE EAT AND DO:

Sauté onion in oil until it starts to brown.

Add tomatoes and sauté another few minutes.

Add dried *kapenta* and cook 5-7 minutes over a medium hot heat

Water may be added if you prefer more gravy.

Add the fish after the onions have started to brown and then add the tomatoes in the last 5 minutes, Enjoy!

When God incorporated meat into our diet, He had special instructions of what could or could not be eaten:

> *And the pig, though it has a split hoof completely divided, does not chew the cud; it is unclean for you. Of all the creatures living in the water of the seas and the streams, you may eat any that have fins and scale (Leviticus 11:7,9).*

We are what we eat. The fact that pigs eat anything they can find, including dirt, while sea food such as shrimp feed on parasites and skin that they pick off dead animals at the bottom of the sea makes them dirty, unhealthy animals. Shrimp is also considered a high cholesterol food. So when we eat these kinds of animals, we are putting in our bodies what they eat, including increasing our cholesterol level.

Protein is one of the most versatile foods because it can come from animals as well as plants like beans and soy. Some of the protein filled exotic protein foods are now being discovered in the western world and yet most of us grew up eating them, just as our forefathers in the Bible did:

> *But you may eat insects if they have legs with joints above their feet so that they can jump. You may also eat all kinds of locusts, all kinds of winged locusts, all kinds of crickets, and all kinds of grasshoppers (Leviticus 11:21-22).*

A smile may cross some of our faces as we reminisce chasing after *mhashu/whiza* (locust), or *shwarra/ishwa* (flying termites). We also might have fond memories of the times we spent with *ambuya tichijuruja majuru* (grandma catching red ants) or her bringing home *macimbi/madora/mahlonza* (mopane worms). According to the U. N. Food and Agriculture Organization, there are many edible insects that are packed with protein, fiber, good fats, and vital minerals, minerals as much if not more than many other food sources such as fish and meat. After *madora* that *mbuya* brought home were dried, they could be cooked and enjoyed as follows:

Madora/macimbi/mahlonza can be soaked or boiled before being cooked:

- 3 cups *madora*
- Salt to taste
- Cayenne pepper to taste
- ½ Onion
- 1 tomato

- 2tbs extra virgin olive oil

While *madora* are boiling, sauté onions and tomatoes into a stew with cayenne pepper to taste

When *madora* are tender, add the stew and cook till ready to eat.

Options to this dish include adding either peanut butter or low-fat cream and cooking till ready to eat. ENJOY!

Fats

Speak to the people of Israel, saying, You shall eat no fat of ox or sheep or goat. The fat of an animal that dies of itself and the fat of one that is torn by beasts may be put to any other use, but on no account shall you eat it (Leviticus 7:23-24)

Some of us remember eating *nyama ine mafuta* (fatted beef) with *muriwo* cooked in just a little bit more generous portions of *mafuta* (fat) and thoroughly enjoying this dish. Little did we know that we were clogging our arteries with extra fat. It is possible that the reason we did not hear of many heart disease cases back then might have been because of our daily active life styles that prevented plaque build-up. Our body actually makes all the fat we need, including cholesterol; therefore, any fat and cholesterol we eat is extra and unnecessary. It is no wonder God commands us not to eat fat. Most of the fats we eat are from added fat when we cook and fry. However, natural occurring fats can be found in foods from animals including eggs, dairy products, and lard. Fat provides us with more sources of energy than carbohydrates. We need fat to help sustain our normal core body temperature while insulating us from the cold and help in the absorption of fat-soluble vitamins A, D, E, and K. Fat allows the proper function of cells and the nervous system, as well as helps us maintain healthy hair and skin.

Fats are divided into unsaturated good fats, saturated bad fats, and trans fats, the worst kind of fats. Unsaturated fats generally come from vegetables and plants and are usually liquid at room temperature. They consist of monounsaturated and polyunsaturated fats. Unsaturated fats are the healthiest of the fats because they have been shown to help reduce levels of bad cholesterol lowering our good cholesterol. Monounsaturated fats are liquid at room temperature but begin to solidify at cold temperatures. This type of fat is preferable to other types of fats and can be found in plants like olives, olive oil, nuts, peanut oil, canola oil and avocados.

An example of polyunsaturated fats is the Omega-3 fatty acids. These are also part of "essential" fatty acid, which means they are critical for our health but cannot be manufactured by our bodies. Good sources of omega-3 fatty acids include cold-water fish, flax seed, soy, safflower, sesame, corn, cottonseed, and walnuts. These fatty acids may reduce the risk of coronary heart disease, fight inflammation, protect the brain and nervous system and also boost our immune systems.

WE ARE WHAT WE EAT AND DO:

Saturated fats are derived from animal products such as meat, dairy and eggs. But they are also found in some plant-based sources such as coconut, palm and palm kernel oils. These fats are solid at room temperature. Saturated fats are considered bad because they directly raise the bad cholesterol levels.

Trans fats or hydrogenated fats are actually unsaturated fats that are created by industrial processing, by adding hydrogen to liquid vegetable oils to make them more solid. This is done to extend the shelf life of processed foods, typically cookies, cakes, fries and donuts. Trans fats are the worse and should be avoided by all means as they also can clog arteries.

Cholesterol is part of fat that our body already makes and is also found in our blood stream from the food we eat and from what our cells already make. The body produces cholesterol because it helps make the outer coating of our body cells, the bile acids that work to digest food in the intestine, as well as Vitamin D and hormones, like estrogen and testosterone. So even if we eat a completely cholesterol-free diet, our body can regulate cholesterol production, needed to properly function.

Cholesterol is a waxy, fat-like substance that comes as low-density lipoproteins (LDL), the bad cholesterol and high-density lipoproteins (HDL), and the good cholesterol. Having healthy levels of both types of lipoproteins is important for body function.

What happens then when we eat fat? Only mechanical digestion takes place in the mouth when we chew and swallow fat. When the fat reaches our stomach, it is broken down by the churning of the stomach muscles before it is delivered to the small intestine as chyme. When the chyme enters the upper portion of the small intestine, the hormones signal the gallbladder to push bile made by the liver into the small intestine. Fat is not water soluble; therefore, bile emulsifies it to help with the digestive process. At the same time, the pancreas secretes chemicals and enzymes that further help break down fat into fatty acids and monoglycerides. These smaller fat particles are then able to pass through the small intestine, converted to triglycerides, and combine with cholesterol and other chemicals so it can travel through the lymph vessels to the bloodstream. **Just like all the final fat products of excess carbohydrates and protein, fatty acids from fat are also stored in the liver till they are needed and processed for energy. Any excess fat also ends up being stored as fat in our body parts.**

However, at the end of the day, a good fat is still a fat in terms of calories. So it is very important to read labels, keeping in mind that food labels proudly stating 0g trans fats, does not transform it into a health food. It might mean that the hydrogenated fat has been replaced by another kind of fat, often a saturated tropical fat, which may or may not be more beneficial.

What I now know

In this chapter what I found most interesting is:

_____

_____

_____

_____

_____

~~~~

From this chapter I intend to do the following toward healthier eating:

_____

_____

_____

_____

_____

CHAPTER SEVENTEEN

REVELATION: ZVAKARATIDZWA

Then God said, "I give you every seed-bearing plant on the face of the whole earth and every tree that has fruit with seed in it. They will be yours for food (Genesis 1:29)

It is very important to know Who we are and where we come from. We come from the Creator of everything on earth and beyond who said everything was good after He created it. In the beginning God provided us with a vegetarian diet. Later, He allowed us to eat meat. Even as He did so, this allowance came with restrictions such as not eating the blood of the meat, certain kinds of meat, and certain parts of meat such as fat (See APPENDIX E for a list of foods in the Bible and where they are mentioned). As we go on, the Bible instructs us that as we give thanks for the food in front of us, not to overeat. All this is done to preserve us and keep us healthy to live a long happy, prosperous life in Him. God created us to reflect Him:

So God created mankind in his own image, in the image of God he created them; male and female he created them (Genesis 1: 27).

WE ARE WHAT WE EAT AND DO:

He made us in His own image, meaning He wanted us to reflect Him. By this we know for sure that He knows and wants what is best for us and would do anything to help us reflect His image. God is also very much concerned for our well-being. He desires to provide for us, and He loves us to the point that He sent His only Son to save us. But what does being created in His image mean to us? It means that God wants to share the same qualities He has such as intelligence, strength, patience, diligence, discernment, and having the capacity to think rationally. We need these characteristics to be successful in keeping God's statutes and in making the right decisions at the right time for our well-being and health. If, however, we are not aware, the devil comes to steal, kill, and destroy us:

> Be alert and of sober mind. Your enemy the devil prowls around like a roaring lion looking for someone to devour (1 Peter 5:8).

We are not and should not be constrained to this world. We should always be aware of our surroundings, not accepting that which is not of God. We should also be capable of resisting what is not good and healthy. We should not act on instinct but should be able to control our natural drives for a higher purpose.

When it comes to food, this drive can overcome some of us. We are surrounded by so many tantalizing commercials offering us to try empty calorie filled new meal. When we go shopping, we often see groceries offer buy one and get one free deals and we are tempted because it seems this will save us money. We have so far been presented with what is around us, what is on our plates and how to use it successfully, but temptations can be our stumbling block unless we put our faith in God:

> *No temptation has overtaken you that is not common to man. God is faithful, and he will not let you be tempted beyond your ability, but with the temptation he will also provide the way of escape, that you may be able to endure it (1 Corinthians 10:13).*

Yes, God is gracious enough that He gave us free will. We all have the ability to choose what we do, how we do it, and when as well as with whom we do it. There is plenty of healthy food that God created for us, but let us not be boastful about our free will and be blind to what and how much we should eat and how we should behave:

> *"I have the right to do anything," you say—but not everything is beneficial. "I have the right to do anything"— but I will not be mastered by anything. You say, "Food for the stomach and the stomach for food, and God will destroy them both..." (1 Corinthians 6: 12- 13a).*

WE ARE WHAT WE EAT AND DO:

Therefore, to preserve God's image, we have to reflect Him in all His glory and goodness. God exudes health and excellence. That said, we have to present our bodies as acceptable to Him who created us. We can only do this by following His living Word no matter what the world has to offer us. Again:

> Therefore I urge you, brethren, by the mercies of God, to present your bodies a living and holy sacrifice, acceptable to God, which is your spiritual service of worship. And do not be conformed to this world, but be transformed by the renewing of your mind, so that you may prove what the will of God is, that which is good and acceptable and perfect (Romans 2:1-2).

There are some Biblical principles that we can follow in order to live a healthier life according to God's plan. Basically, God wants us to eat the foods that He created for us. With that in mind, we should not alter God's design of this food. Last but not least, we should not let any food or drink become our God. Throughout the Bible, the Word emphasizes the importance of proportionality, variety, moderation; therefore, we should apply this to maintain a nutritious diet. God's laws are intended to bless and benefit us spiritually, physically, and socially, and He desires for us to be healthy even in this fallen world. That is why He provided us with guidelines and commandments. If we abide by them, God will provide success in everything in our lives, including health:

146

He said, "If you listen carefully to the voice of the LORD your God and do what is right in his eyes, if you pay attention to his commands and keep all his decrees, I will not bring on you any of the diseases I brought on the Egyptians, for I am the LORD, who heals you" (Exodus 15:26).

God promises to meet all our needs, but we need to be open to scrutiny and self-examination. We should also be ready to accept that which is exposed to us for our health betterment:

Search me, God, and know my heart; test me and know my anxious thoughts. And see if there be any hurtful way in me, and lead me in the everlasting way (Psalm 139 23-24).

Our health improvement will also be established when we focus on God, for when all is said and done, it is not the food or lack of it that makes us Holy:

But food does not bring us near to God; we are no worse if we do not eat, and no better if we do (1 Corinthians 8:8).

One definite affirmation that we get from the Bible is that it tells us:

I praise you, for I am fearfully and wonderfully made. Wonderful are your works; my soul knows it very well (Psalm 139:14).

WE ARE WHAT WE EAT AND DO:

In conclusion, there are some things to think about as we compare cultural differences between Zimbabwe and a place like the United States, in which some Zimbabweans might have settled. Some of us cannot help but chuckle at the irony of life between the haves and the have-nots. In the U.S, Americans who are less financially fortunate are more likely to eat less healthy than less fortunate Zimbabweans in Zimbabwe. For instance, taking all the factors previously discussed such as limited time, financial constraints, access, and a bunch of hungry kids into consideration, an American is more likely to buy pizza and a 2-liter bottle of coke for dinner. Meanwhile back home, a less financially fortunate Zimbabwean would make time and be more likely to buy some fresh vegetables, beans or lacto, and *sadza* will be ready for dinner. On the flip side, those who are more financial fortunate here in the U.S are more likely to buy and cook at home or order in healthier food, while back home the same are more likely to buy fast food, as it is seen as a luxury only a few can afford. As we now know, most fast foods are not as healthy as fresh cooked foods.

God wants to give us all a new look from inside and out. Therefore,

Pakupedzisira hamadzngu zvose zvazvokwadi, zvose
zvinokudzwa, zvose zvakarurama, zvose zvakachena, zvose
zvinidikanwa, zvose zvinorumbidzwa, kana kunaka kupi
nokupi, kana cingarumbidzwa chipi nechipi, fungisisai izvozvo.
Zvinhu izvo zvamakadzidza, nezvamakavona kwandiri,

148

itai izvozvo: Mwari worugare ngaave nemwi (VaFiripi 4:8-9)

Finally, brothers, whatever is true, whatever is noble, whatever is right, whatever is pure, whatever is lovely, whatever is admirable--if anything is excellent or praiseworthy--think about such things. Whatever you have learned or received or heard from me, or seen in me--put it into practice. And the God of peace will be with you (Philippians 4: 8-9).

What I now know

In this chapter what I found most interesting is:

_____

_____

_____

_____

_____

~~~~

From this chapter I intend to do the following toward healthier eating:

_____

_____

_____

_____

_____

HEALTHY WAYS TO PRESERVE FOOD NUTRIENTS

Action	Rationale
Keep fruits & vegetables cool.	Enzymes in food begin to degrade vitamins once the fruit or vegetable is picked. Chilling reduces this process. Refrigerate fresh produce (except for potatoes, tomatoes, onions, and bananas) until they are consumed.
Refrigerate food in moisture-proof, air-tight containers.	Nutrients keep best at temperatures near freezing, at high humidity, and away from air.
Trim, peel, cut fruits & vegetables minimally, enough to remove rotten or inedible parts.	Oxygen breaks down vitamins faster when more surface is exposed. Outer leaves of lettuce and other greens have higher values of vitamins and minerals than the inner, tender leaves or stems. Potato skins and apple skins are higher in vitamins and minerals than the inner parts.
Microwave, steam, or use a pan or wok with very small amounts of fat and a tight-fitting lid to cook vegetables.	More nutrients are retained when there is less contact with water and shorter cooking time. Whenever possible, cook fruits or vegetables in their skins.

Action	Rationale
Minimize reheating food.	Prolonged reheating reduces vitamin content.
Do not add fats to vegetables during cooking if you plan to discard the liquid.	Fat-soluble vitamins will be lost in discarded fat. Add fats to vegetables after they are fully cooked and drained.
Do not add baking soda to vegetables to enhance the green color.	Alkalinity destroys much thiamin, and other vitamins.
Store canned foods in a cool place.	Canned foods vary in the amount of nutrients lost, largely because of differences in storage time and temperatures. To get maximal nutritive value from canned goods, serve any liquid packed with the food whenever possible.

APPENDIX: B

HEALTH BENEFITS OF HONEY

Health Issue	Benefits
Related to overall nutrition	Healthiest sweetener even can be used by those with Type-2 diabetes
	Due to its low Glycemic index it is NOT the same as white sugar or artificial sweeteners - helps the body regulate blood sugar levels.
	Contains an array of vitamins and minerals: niacin, riboflavin, pantothenic acid, calcium, copper, iron, magnesium, manganese, phosphorus, potassium and zinc
Related to stomach (1-2 tbs before heavy meals)	As antimicrobial agent that benefits the entire digestive tract.
	Has enzyme (glucose oxidase) that produces small amounts of hydrogen peroxide that can treat gastritis.
	Neutralizes gas, which often occurs with overeating
Related to respiratory Cough-2tsp-buckwheat Allergies-1tbs local honey	Helps with coughs, especially at night cough allowing proper sleep
	Helps with sore throats and upper airways-fight infection and soothe membranes For allergies caused by local bee-carried pollens

Health Issue	Benefits
Related to beauty and skin	Has drying properties and able to reach deep tissue. Due to its antimicrobial and antifungal can be used for skin infections. Applied directly to skin or in a dressing and change every 24 to 48 hours. When used directly, apply 15 mL to 30 mL every 12 to 48 hours, and covered with sterile gauze and bandages or a polyurethane dressing. Has natural antiseptic, antibacterial and antimicrobial properties. These properties help clean wounds and cuts keep wounds and cuts free from infection, reduce odor and pus, lessen pain and promote speedy healing.
	For minor burn, apply to the affected area. Within sometime, you will feel relief from the burning and itching sensation and pain. Apply honey on minor burn several times a day for several days to promote fast healing.
	Ultimate ingredient to use for healthy and glowing skin. For blemishes, apply a little bit of honey directly on the affected area before going to bed for several days. This will give the skin all night to absorb the honey's medicinal properties. Wash it off the next morning with lukewarm water and soon you will have clear and glowing skin.
	Can also treat other skin conditions like eczema, ringworm and psoriasis, reduce skin inflammation and relieve dryness.

Health Issue	Benefits
Related to hair/scalp	For chronic seborrheic dermatitis and dandruff- apply honey diluted with warm water to problem areas and leave it on for 3 hours before rinsing with warm water and continue weekly thereafter for 6 months
Related to antioxidation (1tbs) With ACV with mother	Full of antioxidants- drinking a glass of lukewarm water with honey and lemon juice on an empty stomach, first thing in the morning. This helps with detoxification, cleansing the liver, removing toxins, and flushing fat out of the body, thereby promoting weight loss
Related to Cancer	Has tumor-fighting properties, and may help prevent colon cancer
Related to weight loss	Contains vitamins, minerals and amino acids, work together to promote fat and cholesterol metabolism, which in turn helps maintain body weight and prevents obesity. Detoxification also helps promote weight loss
Related to sleep	Is a fat-digesting carbohydrate that stimulates the release of insulin and allows tryptophan – a compound that makes us sleepy) to enter the brain easily. A glass of warm milk with honey before going to bed. Both honey and milk are tryptophan-containing foods.
Related to energy and performance (1 tbs of honey before workout or in the morning)	Helps reduced muscle fatigue by boosting performance and endurance levels and reduce muscle fatigue. Provides sustained energy to the body, also maintaining glycogen levels during performance and improve recovery time,

APPENDIX: C

COMMON AILMENTS, FUNCTIONAL FOODS, AND DIETARY SUPPLEMENTS

Purpose	Functional Foods and Dietary Supplements
Beauty- skin, hair, nails	Vitamin C, D, E, Biotin, vitamin B-complex Greet tea extract Aloe Honey Cucumbers
Diabetes- Blood Sugar	Vitamins: D, B1- thiamine, B3- niacin, B6 pyridoxine Antioxidants Chromium Coenzyme Q10 Garlic Cucumbers Apple cider vinegar with the mother
Neuropathy	Chromium Cinnamon Zinc Garlic Ginseng
Headache	Peppermint
Swelling	Tomatoes Cucumbers Watermelon

Purpose	Functional Foods and Dietary Supplements
Arthritis Bones/ Joint	Antioxidants: Green tea, green leafy vegetables, berries Calcium Magnesium Glucosamine Sulfate Chondroitin Omega 3 fatty acids Turmeric Vitamin D
Cognitive health- Memory/Fatigue	Omega 3 fatty acids Vitamin C, D Vitamin B 12 and (6) folic acid Acetyl-L Carnitine N- acetyl-L-cysteine SAM-e Tumeric CoQ10- Magnesium Watermelon
Stress/Tension	Green leafy vegetables Pumpkin seeds Chamomile tea
Digestive health	Probiotics- Lactobacillus acidophilus Apple cider vinegar with the mother Ginger Peppermint Prunes Vitamin D Vitamin B 6 Magnesium

Purpose	Functional Foods and Dietary Supplements
Heart health	Omega 3 fatty acids- salmon, sardine, tuna, raw almonds Coenzyme Q10 Magnesium Vitamin B complex Flax seed
Cholesterol	Red yeast rice Flax seed Cinnamon Garlic Oats
Immune health	Antioxidants: Green tea, green leafy vegetables, berries
Anti-inflammatory	Antioxidants: Green tea, green leafy vegetabless, berries Fish, nuts, seeds, beans Curry (turmeric), basil, rosemary, ginger Whole grains (highest fiber) High ORAC foods Omega- 3 fatty acids (DHA & EPA) Olive oil
Antioxidants/Cancer prevention	Green Tea Berries Green leafy vegetables Vitamin A, C, E Selenium Whole grains (highest fiber) Omega- 3 fatty acids (DHA & EPA) Milk thistle Vitamin D

Purpose	Functional Foods and Dietary Supplements
Pain	Vitamin D
	Cayenne
	Ginger
	Turmeric
	Rosemary
	Green tea
Menopause	Vitamin B 6 & 12 folic, D, E
	Calcium
	Soy
Men's health	Saw palmetto
Children's health	Calcium
	Iron
	Fluoride
	Vitamin D
	Choline
Prenatal health	Folic
	Calcium
	Iron
	Omega 3 fatty acids
	Vitamin C, D

APPENDIX: D

FOODS MENTIONED IN THE BIBLE (Fairchild)

Seasonings, Spices and Herbs

Anise (Matthew 23:23)

Coriander (Exodus 16:31; Numbers 11:7)

Cinnamon (Exodus 30:23; Revelation 18:13)

Cumin (Isaiah 28:25; Matthew 23:23)

Dill (Matthew 23:23)

Garlic (Numbers 11:5)

Mint (Matthew 23:23; Luke 11:42)

Mustard (Matthew 13:31)

Rue (Luke 11:42)

Salt (Ezra 6:9; Job 6:6)

Grains

Barley (Deuteronomy 8:8; Ezekiel 4:9)

Bread (Genesis 25:34; 2 Samuel 6:19; 16:1; Mark 8:14)

Corn (Matthew 12:1; - refers to "grain" such as wheat or barley)

Flour (2 Samuel 17:28; 1 Kings 17:12)

Millet (Ezekiel 4:9)

Spelt (Ezekiel 4:9)

Unleavened Bread (Genesis 19:3; Exodus 12:20)

Wheat (Ezra 6:9; Deuteronomy 8:8)

Fruits and Nuts

Apples (Song of Solomon 2:5)

Almonds (Genesis 43:11; Numbers 17:8)

Dates (2 Samuel 6:19; 1 Chronicles 16:3)

Figs (Nehemiah 13:15; Jeremiah 24:1-3)

Grapes (Leviticus 19:10; Deuteronomy 23:24)

Melons (Numbers 11:5; Isaiah 1:8)

Olives (Isaiah 17:6; Micah 6:15)

Pistachio Nuts (Genesis 43:11)

Pomegranates (Numbers 20:5; Deuteronomy 8:8)

Raisins (Numbers 6:3; 2 Samuel 6:19)

Sycamore Fruit (Psalm 78:47; Amos 7:14)

Vegetables and Legumes

Beans (2 Samuel 17:28; Ezekiel 4:9)

Cucumbers (Numbers 11:5)

Gourds (2 Kings 4:39)

Leeks (Numbers 11:5)

Lentils (Genesis 25:34; 2 Samuel 17:28; Ezekiel 4:9)

Onions (Numbers 11:5)

Dairy

Butter (Proverbs 30:33)

Cheese (2 Samuel 17:29; Job 10:10)

Curds (Isaiah 7:15)

Milk (Exodus 33:3; Job 10:10; Judges 5:25)

Fish

Matthew 15:36

John 21:11-13

Fowl

Partridge (1 Samuel) 26:20; Jeremiah 17:11)

Pigeon (Genesis 15:9; Leviticus 12:8)

Quail (Psalm 105:40)

Dove (Leviticus 12:8)

Animal Meats

Calf (Proverbs 15:17; Luke 15:23)

Goat (Genesis 27:9)

Lamb (2 Samuel 12:4)

Oxen (1 Kings 19:21)

Sheep (Deuteronomy 14:4)

Venison (Genesis 27:7)

Miscellaneous

Eggs (Job 6:6; Luke 11:12)

Grape Juice (Numbers 6:3)

Honey (Exodus 33:3; Deuteronomy 8:8; Judges 14:8-9)

Locust (Mark 1:6)

Olive Oil (Ezra 6:9; Deuteronomy 8:8)

Vinegar (Ruth 2:14; John 19:29)

Wine (Ezra 6:9; John 2:1-10

APPENDIX: E

BIBLIOGRAPHY

Amazing benefits of honey. (2014). Retrieved from
http://www.benefits-of-honey.com/

Anorexia nervosa and bulimia nervosa (n.d). Retrieved from
http://www.medschool.pitt.edu/somsa/Anorexia.html

Beattie, L. & Barnes, L. (2014). Wild or farmed fish: What's better?
Retrieved from
http://www.sparkpeople.com/resource/nutrition_articles.a
sp?id=1282

Benefits of pasture-based and grass fed farming (2014).
Retrieved from
http://animalwelfareapproved.org/consumers/healthbenefi
ts/

Berardi, J (2013). Breakfast: Not really the most important meal of
the day Retrieved from
http://www.huffingtonpost.com/johnberardiphd/breakfast
health_b_4436439.html

Braggs (2012). How to use the powerful health qualities of natural
apple cider vinegar. Retrieved from
http://bragg.com/books/acv_excerpt.html

Daniels, C. (2011). Alpha lipoic Acid vs. conjugated linoleic acid
Retrieved from http://www.livestrong.com/article/475972-
alpha-lipoic-acid-vs-conjugated-linoleic-acid/

Dickens, C. (1859). *A tale of two cities*. London, UK: Chapman and
Hall

Donatelle, R. J. (2011). *Health: The basics* (Green ed.). Boston, MA:
Benjamin Cummings.

Dr Oz show(2011). 7-Day miracle plan to boost your metabolism.
Retrieved from

Fairchild, M (2014). Foods of the Bible. Retrieved from

http://christianity.about.com/od/biblefactsandlists/qt/foods
ofthebible.htm

FDA (2013). Once baby arrives: Food safety for mom-to-be.
Retrieved from
http://www.fda.gov/food/resourcesforyou/healtheducators
/ucm089629.htm

GMO Project (2013). Retrieved from
http://www.nongmoproject.org/learn-more/

Grosvenor, M. B., & Smolin, L. A. (2012). *Visualizing nutrition:
Everyday choices* (2nd ed.). Hoboken, NJ: Wiley.

Herrington, D. (2012). 10 health benefits of honey. Retrieved from
http://www.care2.com/greenliving/10-health-benefits-of-
honey.html

How do fruits and vegetables lose their nutrients after picking?
Retrieved from http://www.livestrong.com/article/447449-
how-do-fruits-and-vegetables-lose-their-nutrients-after-
picking/

Institute for Responsible Technology. (2013). 10 Reasons to avoid
GMOs. Retrieved from
http://www.responsibletechnology.org/10-Reasons-to-
Avoid-GMOs

Institute of Food Research. (2014). Retrieved from
http://www.ifr.ac.uk/

Loughlin, J. (1907). St. Ambrose. In the Catholic Encyclopedia.
New York: Robert Appleton Company. Retrieved New
Advent: http://www.newadvent.org/cathen/01383c.htm

Martin L. J. (2014). What researchers are learning about honey's
possible health benefits. Retrieved from
http://www.webmd.com/diet/features/medicinal-uses-of-
honey

Mercola, J. (2013). Intermittent fasting — More a lifestyle than a
diet. Retrieved from
http://fitness.mercola.com/sites/fitness/archive/2013/06/28/i
ntermittent-fasting-health-benefits.aspx

Mitchell, H. H., Hamilton, T. S., Steggerda, F. R., & Bean, H. W. (1945). The chemical composition of the adult human body and its bearing on the biochemistry of growth *J. Biol. Chem. 158: 625-637.*

National Cancer Institute. (2010). Chemicals in meat cooked at high temperatures and cancer risk. Retrieved from http://www.cancer.gov/cancertopics/factsheet/Risk/cooked -meats

Nutritious effects of food processing. (2014). Retrieved from http://nutritiondata.self.com/topics/processing

Oxford Dictionary. (2014). Diet. Retrieved from http://www.oxforddictionaries.com/definition/english/diet ?q=diet

Polland, M. (2009). *The Omnivore's Dilemma: The Secretes behind what you eat.* Penguin Group: New York, NY.

Robinson, J (20214). *Pasture perfect: how you can benefit from choosing meat, eggs, and dairy products from grass-fed animals.* Vashon, Washington: Vashon Island Press

Russell, R. *(1996). What the Bible says about healthy living* Regal Books: Ventura CA

Sustainable livestock husbandry. (2014). Retrieved from http://www.sustainabletable.org/248/sustainable-livestock-husbandry

Top 10 Home remedies. (2014). Retrieved from http://www.top10homeremedies.com/

USDA. (2013). Cutting boards and food safety. Retrieved from http://www.fsis.usda.gov/wps/portal/fsis/topics/food-safety-education/get-answers/food-safety-fact-sheets/safe-food-handling/cutting-boards-and-food-safety/ct_INDEX

What are the Benefits of "Free-Range? (2014). Retrieved from http://www.sunrisefarm.net/newsarticles/benefitsoffreeran ge.html

The Oz Show (2013). 7-day miracle plan to boost your

Metabolism http://www.doctoroz.com/videos/7-day-miracle-plan-boost-your-metabolism?page=2

Wardlaw, G. M., & Smith, A. M. (2011). *Contemporary nutrition* (8th ed.). New York, NY: McGraw-Hill

Zelman, K, M. (20154). The truth about 6 meals a day for weight loss: Can eating more frequently help you lose weight? Retrieved from http://www.webmd.com/diet/features/truth-about-6-meals-day-weight-loss